The Secret of Health

by

Richard Lynch

UNITY BOOKS
UNITY VILLAGE, MISSOURI

Contents

The Secret of Health

The healing message is the very essence of Christianity. Throughout the Gospel story Jesus practiced it as the most important branch of His ministry. He sent His disciples forth to "preach" and to "heal." In the early days of the Christian religion healing seems never to have been separated from the idea of teaching. It was the prominent characteristic of the ministry of primitive Christianity, and failure to discern its principles is to disregard the most momentous element of Jesus' life and work.

Intelligently understood, healing is concerned with every condition of life and covers all the needs of man. Although we usually think of it in connection with physical health, it applies equally well to our circumstances and affairs. Jesus was a health giver in the fullest sense of the term, a savior who healed the hurts of man, not partially but wholly, in every department of his being.

In this series of articles I shall apply the spiritual principles that He taught to all human problems and prove that the action of Truth results inevitably in a healing demonstration. When we discern the spiritual nature of man and his universe, we rise above material limitations into health and wholeness: health of body, wealth in affairs, and satisfaction of spirit.

To accomplish any definite result the principle back of the manifestation must be understood. Often this requires a complete transformation of thought and an establishment of ideals definite and powerful enough to rebuild the entire attitude toward life. Christianity is both definite and positive, teaching a practical method of spiritual healing to those who clearly see its true meaning.

There is nothing new or startling about spiritual healing. It antedates medical science. We read of it in the history of all nations. Instances of it are recorded throughout the Bible. Jesus did not make the healing law, but He did understand and practice it. Based as it is upon demonstrable principle, when properly employed it is as effective today as it was two thousand years ago.

In the story of Job we read that he suffered long and grievously before the realization came to him that he had been utterly mistaken in his conception of God. "Who is this that hides counsel without knowledge? Therefore I have uttered what I did not understand, things too wonderful for me, which I did not know," was his cry. "Hear, and I will speak; I will question you, and you declare to me. I had heard of thee by the hearing of the ear, but now my eye sees thee." We too have listened to many misinterpretations of our good, marveling that our cries have not been heard and answered and not realizing that it is because we have not understood aright.

When spiritual healing is analyzed it is found to be strictly in accordance with natural law. It is the result of harmony, a finely balanced adjustment between mind and body. When the mind is disordered the equilibrium of the body is disturbed. Mind literally governs the body as a creative coordinator or guide, whose thought activity supervises bodily expression. We all know how it molds the features, showing forth states of discontent or of joyous cheer. As the state of mind is changed the expression alters. Thoughts are published from the housetops of physical aspects and material conditions.

The metaphysician knows that the problem of physical health cannot be treated as an outside condition but that it is a result of thoughts held in consciousness and that by applying correct principles the power of thought can be regulated and constructively applied. Health of mind must inevitably result in health of body. Jesus recognized all the ills of humanity as the effect of erroneous human concepts, and He treated disease, discord, and death through mind and spirit.

As mind is the life of man's body, it is clearly evident that a mind filled with the divine essence of true thought cannot picture forth shadowy creations of error. Jesus, by His marvelous clarity of vision, eliminated the effect of false thinking in others, but His advice was, "Sin no more." We understand the sin that He sought to correct was failure to think in terms of Truth. He performed the cure, but permanent healing was dependent upon the individual himself. Continually He bore witness to the Truth, in which He had found the secret of well-being.

"You will know the truth, and the truth will make you free." Truth is something that is, a positive something that exists. The negative error—a nonentity—lacks existence; it *is not*. Error is the root of disease, the foundation of sickness and inharmonious conditions. As Truth is substituted for error something is supplied in place of the fallacious idea or wrong thought.

To know the Truth is to identify one's individual self with the infinite Father source of all life. The individual self is like a house wired for electricity; the owner by simply turning a switch floods it with light from a great central generating plant that is the source of all the light of a great city. Or the self is like a dry, thirsty field that by means of floodgates communicates with the giant reservoir of a great irrigation system that supplies lifegiving water to all dry, thirsty fields.

God is the infinite source of the one power that is. Man is wired for contacting this power; channeled for its cleansing inflow. As he knows this, identifying himself with the Spirit of life, he opens the floodgates to Truth and sets in operation the divine law of spiritual healing.

Positive, constructive thought keeps the Truth channels open for this free-flowing life of God. Negative, error thought raises barriers and obstructs the healing current. We have all experienced this power of mind to regulate the body, negatively if not positively. Feverish headache, tense muscles, inactive digestion, and restless nerves have resulted from anger, fear, and worry.

9

We have the ability through our thought to change the direction of these attitudes of mind. By substituting faith for fear, love for hate, confidence for doubt, we may demolish the barriers that obstruct the flow of the universal life that is ever seeking to rebuild and repair our organism.

Every true thought has in it some of the life of God, of the one and only reality, of the divine essence of Being. Nothing in the universe possesses a higher therapeutic value. True thinking is the basis of correct expression. God holds man in His consciousness as an ideal or type man. As such man's faculties are eternally perfect; they existed before the organic structure of the body came into manifestation. The perception of this principle, the recognition of an ideal man whose every faculty is spiritual power, must invariably correct all conditions of seeming imperfection.

It is a great mistake to place the physical function on the organ instead of knowing that each function existed in the consciousness of God before the creation of the organ and that it is eternally held there in permanent security. To understand sight and hearing as spiritual ideas, inherent in the principle of Being, is to mold the eyes and ears into responsive organs of expression. As the body idea is God's creation, it must be perfect. If it appears inharmonious or discordant, the trouble lies not in the body but in a wrong idea about it.

Christianity gives us positive ideas; it teaches that God is omnipresent. It conveys to man the consciousness that since he is in Omnipresence, established in it, he is safe and secure. Because this conviction is based upon Truth, it destroys fear. No one who has a firm conviction of safety can be a prey to fear; no one whose heart is filled with "good will toward men" can understand hatred, envy, or jealousy; no one who holds steadfast an image of the divine ideal of perfection can manifest the negativity of ill-health.

There is no reality in anything that changes. Reality is Truth, and Truth is unchangeable. We manifest health only by conforming to the heavenly pattern, the divine design for man's life. In the kingdom of Mind this realization of true wholeness is "at hand," to be demonstrated and enjoyed, but it demands a recognition of the purpose of infinite intelligence in individual expression.

All healing is a matter of consciousness and begins with the mind. Man himself lays the foundations of health and disease by his persistent habits of thought. Many still believe that sickness is something thrust upon them to try their patience and strengthen their faith. But it was never God's will that any person should suffer and remain sick, unhappy, or poor. God's will is always good will; it is unreservedly for a fuller expression of life, physically, mentally, and spiritually.

In the consciousness of man there is a region that is not subject to change. The material body may alter and external conditions may vary. Thoughts, feelings, and environment may change, but there is an entity that has persisted unchanged throughout the individual's conscious existence, "the same yesterday and today, and for ever." It cannot be called material, this intangible, unchangeable, eternal thing. It is Spirit; therefore it cannot be sick, diseased, unhappy, or inharmonious.

When you say "I am" in connection with any of the foregoing, you are uttering an untruth, for all that is of the I AM is divine. I AM is the highest expression of divinity, the name that God claimed as an immortal expression of His omnipotence. Even a glimpse of this eternal idea of an unchanging, undying self that is not and cannot be diseased inspires in one an impulse to externalize its perfection or, as Paul would express it, to "put on the Lord Jesus Christ."

The emanation of Divine Mind is the perfect

idea, and is the Christ within. Realization of this truth compelled Jesus to say, "I am the Son of God." The Spirit of God acclaimed Him: "This is my beloved Son, with whom I am well pleased." This is how man also must affirm the reality of the true self in order to experience the Christ Spirit.

This power which purifies, strengthens, and upholds becomes real only to those who long for it and who open the channels of their cleansed hearts to receive it. It does not come to one who does not really and steadfastly desire it. To those who possess this intuitive consciousness of divine life in the soul, this life must of necessity come into free expression through the body as health, through the mind as harmony, and through the affairs as progress. For a changed consciousness creates for itself a new physical expression or outward condition to harmonize with its altered spiritual viewpoint.

A renewed consciousness transforms the body temple, as a result of spiritual chemistry, into "the beauties of holiness" or wholeness, which comparatively few have understood but which daily become more sought after. Beginning in the mind, health is the normal result of right living, and the basis of right living is right thinking. Permanent healing comes only through a sustained change of thought crystallizing into absolute conviction or belief.

As long as any inharmony remains in the consciousness, any clashing of the human with the divine will, as long as any discordant, unrestrained emotions run riot, true harmony cannot be established. All spiritual healing is a restoration of harmony between man and his divine Source, which becomes manifest as the self is continually lifted up to the divine standard. To perceive that all man's powers and all his faculties, being in Divine Mind, are always perfect and that the body registers our beliefs about these powers and faculties is the secret of healing. We redeem our body as we get the true insight into all its potentialities.

The most important question in each life should be "What must I do to be saved"—from the sin of wrong thinking? How can I erase the errors of race thought? How can I free myself from subconscious material beliefs, of which the body is miscreated? How can I effect the radical change in mental status and establish the mode of thought that will pluck from the mind the deeply rooted origin of disease?

In order that the consciousness may be charged with God thought the heart must be free from negative, destructive sense emotions, the nerves must be poised and centered in the Christ ideal, the vision must be fixed upon the true reality of the perfection that is God. A positive belief in the truth of all this and a steadfast determination to bring it into visible expression will enter and possess the consciousness if you will allow it. The same mind that healed diseased bodies, refusing to recognize even the appearance of evil or error and having no realization of sickness or death, the mind "which was also in Christ Jesus," will fill you with the warmth and light of its life, its love, and its Truth, and make of you "a new creature."

We are working to make humanity aware that it is not a debased and fallen race but one capable of limitless expansion and upward progress. To become aware of this ourselves and to help others to become aware of it is the purpose of our work. Never before, since man lost the first radiance of the Christian religion, has there been such an assurance of the possibilities of man for advancement. If instead of shrinking from the responsibilities of life we assume our share and do our part in awakening the race to a realization of its privileges and powers, we have gained the inmost essence of religion. In this bearing witness to the Truth we shall find the secret of healing.

Where Health Begins

Spiritual health begins with a conscious knowledge of Truth principles and is the basis of all physical soundness. It is an active expression of God energy, and mind is the motive power that sets physical forces in operation either for good or for ill. Through his higher understanding man may become the conquering lord of every activity of his body. By means of his divine intelligence he may make for himself a superhuman law by which he can overcome weariness, disease, and old age. As he bears and controls the "image of the man of dust" he may also "bear the image of the man of heaven" and see God in his flesh.

Health of body as an expression of spiritual health is a normal state, and it is naturally ours unless it is blocked up by fears or wrong beliefs

16

that produce disease. When such irritations are removed and the interference with natural health is taken away, the disease disappears, although its permanent disappearance is dependent upon keeping the consciousness free from the return of disturbing conditions.

This spiritual health which we are all longing to express is an actual departure from mortal thought so absolute and complete that it is impossible ever to think on that basis again. It is a renewal of consciousness, and identification with the source of our being. It is the result of consciously knowing the principles of life and remaining continually aware of the divine presence. When such a change of thought occurs and we see the real of ourself or of another—the true existence as it is in God consciousness—we have attained the spiritual health that is certain to manifest itself in permanent physical healing.

Man is a manifestation of human consciousness in varying degrees, from the simple to the complex, each individual standing as the personification of his own dominant idea. His consciousness projected outward is aware of a world of concrete form and externalized matter, an objective universe, and the connecting link between the subjective and the objective is the mind.

17

The mind is made up of those things of which we are conscious or aware by means of perception. The individual consciousness is developed by thought and colored by whatever persistently dominates the mental activity. The mind as it thinks is continually choosing or rejecting. As you think you become; therefore your consciousness is the creator of your world, as you are the creator of your consciousness.

Living in a material world and through self-interest keying ourselves to its tone of superficiality and sophistication, we are apt to become so concerned with tangible things that we fail to value the invisible and intangible realm that lies all about and within us. We are aware only of those fixed memories of the race which have registered as inharmony, unhappiness, disease, and death, which have descended to us through heredity.

I do not say, as many seem to do, that a weak, sickly body indicates that its possessor has deliberately dwelt upon sickness and disease, literally thinking them into existence, or that certain diseases are the instantaneous creations of suddenly acquired concepts. They are the expression of modes of thought and feeling held in mind until with the lapse of time they have become an integral part of the consciousness.

When people assure me that they have never even thought of many of the ills that come upon them, I try to explain that such manifestations positively prove the presence in their consciousness of negative "germs," such as destructive sparks of fear or worry, envy or jealousy, criticism or condemnation, hatred or revenge, which originate in human beliefs and opinions. These continue to be expressed, to be "bodied forth" in physical form, until people learn to control and nullify them. People have become slaves to these misconceptions and must remain in bondage until they can look past sense impressions and close their ears to echoes of subconscious racial beliefs.

Why do tormenting conditions surround us and irritating pains disturb us? How do we account for the sickness and trouble that remain in the world to sadden us? The answer has long been with us, but we have not yet understood that God's plan includes none of these. Jesus would marvel today at our poverty and disease. He would expect to find a broader vision among us as a result of our increased knowledge and manifestation of Truth. He would be astonished to find that the intelligence that performs modern miracles is not universally associated with the one Intelligence. His own vision of divine perfection was so vivid that

He could heal even the lives of others because He could see so clearly, far above and beyond their human, material beliefs.

It should be just as simple a matter to manifest health as its opposite, yet apparently the contrary is true. There are some minds that have so vivid a consciousness of good that all else is lost sight of or relegated to the background of their life, but they are in the minority. New habits are hard to acquire; yet it is quite possible so to change the consciousness through scientific thinking that it will be elevated beyond the plane of the average mind, to the realm of the superconscious or God mind. This infinite consciousness is the "stronghold" to which the Psalmist says we may flee at any time and find safe refuge from the limitations of human consciousness with its inhibitions and complexes that hamper our freedom.

When we understand that the subconscious mind does not reason but works automatically according to the promptings of the conscious mind, the way to re-educate and renew it becomes plainly evident. As it works without discrimination and reproduces whatever has been gathered and communicated to it, it is quite possible for any person who really and earnestly makes the effort to direct its manifestation in his material world.

The one infallible way of dealing with the operations of the subconscious mind is in accordance with a principle that psychology calls substitution. It is no recent discovery; it has been taught for centuries in Christianity as repentance ("unto forgiveness of sins") or the process of being "born anew." This all conveys the idea of changing the mind, for unless the mind is changed it cannot be renewed or the life transformed. A wrong thought must be changed by the substitution of a true or right thought in its place.

The psychological principle of substitution implies much less than Christian law of repentance, for it is impossible to change the consciousness through will power and autosuggestion. If a person is afraid, he cannot free himself of fear just because he decides to substitute a constructive thought in place of one that is destructive. He must *receive* a positive idea in place of a negative belief.

What does psychology know of love other than as human affection? Christianity is an insight into things as they are, and it informs us: "forms within" our consciousness one of the eternal verities, which is love. Man is forever "in" the love of God, therefore he can readily substitute a positive reality of protective care in the place of fear, which is a false belief of the race.

Psychology regards substitution as replacement, that is, putting something in the place of something else. The repentance of Christianity indicates a "turning about." Our body is a defenseless reproduction of beliefs stored in the subconscious mind, and we find ourselves governed by them unless we learn to control them. They blur our spiritual vision and distort the real or living image of our divine sonship. Often we find ourselves viewing life as a negative picture; that is, a reversed one, as in photography, dark showing for light and light for dark.

In printing a picture the negative is "turned about," and that is just what we must do in stamping our ideas of life with positive realities. We must reverse the negative and see the infinite design in its proper colors. We cannot mix light and darkness; neither can we think Truth and error at the same time. Light blots out darkness; Truth dispels error. "When the perfect comes, the imperfect will pass away."

The heart that is filled with love for humanity has no room for individual hatreds. The life devoted to service has no time for idleness and the mischief it engenders. The consciousness replete with positive ideas of omnipotent good cannot entertain the negative thoughts that produce such destruction in the body and affairs.

I do not say it is possible to live amid present-day conditions with no comprehension or recognition of their presence. But there is a way of looking at life sanely, a way that is wholesome and healthy, a sound, normal way that regards disease as unnatural and abnormal. Such a view is not blind to the morbid, diseased conditions that exist in the world, nor is it indifferent to their tragic effects upon men and women, but it sees them as shadows that may be dissipated by the light of Truth. It substitutes light for darkness, health for sickness, life for death.

There are comparatively few who realize that perfect, normal health is not just freedom from weak hearts, aching muscles, disordered stomachs, and other functional disturbances but that it is a harmonious coordination of spirit, mind, and body. To many it is news to learn that mental and spiritual health have a decisive effect upon the outer physical condition. But the keynote of health is sounded in the Christian religion for a logical reason: because its Founder was a man of authoritative spirit, of pure mind, and of strong body.

Radiations of spirit must be "pressed out" through the individual mind into bodily expression. Mind working through consciousness is the creative force back of all physical health and strength. The process moves in an endless circle. The radiant energy of Spirit rouses the consciousness to action and creates physical vitality; this in turn reacts to reinforce mental energy. Cause and effect are strangely intermingled, therefore balance must be maintained.

Health is God activity, the expression of God energy. It must begin with that "something" within, the health of Spirit, to be unfolded, drawn forth, and employed. Health is an eternal verity, something which *is*, an expression of divine intelligence of which each individual is a part. The more man draws upon this unfailing inexhaustible mind source the more he sets it into activity and the healthier he becomes.

Sunshine is the expression of the sun's light vibrations, with no shadows intervening. So health is the light of Spirit, freed and streaming into expression. It must be manifested by the liberation in consciousness of the perfect conception of wholeness. As repressions of human thought and race belief are released, infinite Energy accomplishes its perfect result.

Jesus taught that except a person be born again he cannot enter the kingdom of God; also that He

Himself was the Resurrection and the life by virtue of His complete regeneration. It is evident that all who are reborn must become that which He became, the Christ. The rebirth He spoke of is a mind process; one that involves a daily "crossing out" or crucifixion of erroneous concepts and a resurrection into that true state of consciousness which is the Christ Mind. It is the entrance into an entirely new existence, with different experiences and changed ideas. Health begins by the discovery in ourselves of the immaculate conception of the Christ idea, which is the Truth of man. To practice the principle that "I and the Father are one" is to awaken within the soul the Christ or God self. With this rebirth comes the conviction of that spiritual well-being which is the beginning of all health.

The Personalization of Health

It has always been the tendency of man to believe in a higher power. Historically this tendency can be traced back through ancient languages and literature as far as thought reaches. No tribe or nation has been found destitute of such a belief. Because every person has always been aware, even though dimly, of "abysmal deeps of personality" and because he has seen, even though "in a mirror, darkly," undeveloped capabilities of energy and power, he should feel conclusive proof of one stupendous truth: that behind the finite personality there lies an infinite or perfect personality, a great reservoir of power waiting to be released through human channels.

Carlyle once called great men "living light-fountains: natural luminaries, shining by the gift of

truth and shedding their radiance upon all souls."
How marvelously this describes one who lived on
this human plane nineteen hundred years ago and
who was to become the most outstanding figure of
all time. We have but a brief record of His life;
notes of words that fell from His lips on a few
occasions; fragments of His teaching and achievements as related by four different men. But the
character of Jesus makes Him the most universal
and significant figure in the history of the world.

How the personality of Jesus dominated every
incident! As a child conversing with learned men in
the Temple, as a friend sorrowing over the spiritual
blindness of the people of Jerusalem, as a teacher
inspiring His followers, as a healer of lack, want,
and disease, as a leader causing hearts to burn
within by the fire of His eloquence and holding
multitudes spellbound by the very magnetism of
His presence, lighting the way for millions, through
dark centuries of ignorant skepticism, overshadow-
ing literature and art and drawing all men unto
Him by a personality that He "lifted up" through
experience with life's realities.

There is no greater or more important work for
you in the universe than the discovery of your real
self, the self that is your character or the result of
your conviction about yourself as a personality;

because this positive conviction about the real self constitutes true healing. When you come into a consciousness of who and what you really are, your health, your place in life, your supply, and your success inevitably unfold. As there is no permanent achievement apart from it, you can see how important it is to solve this great mystery of your own personality.

In Eastern philosophy there is a tendency to efface or destroy the thought of self. In India the belief is current that the more man erases himself the closer he approaches the Infinite. This attempt at self-effacement is often the cause of vague indecision. Weakness, vacillation, and negativity may follow in its wake. Perhaps because the old theology relegated self to the background we may find here the secret of why the past has left few strong, forceful, moving figures and leaders in the ranks of theologians.

In his "Confessions" Augustine speaks of meeting with "himself," and he is amazed that men should go abroad to gaze upon wonders while passing themselves, the crowning wonders, by. "Retire into thyself," he wrote, "for truth dwells in the inner man." Therefore man's sole business should be to discover that hidden wonder, himself, and set the "I" free.

The Latin word *persona* was used to designate the mask worn by an actor in ancient Greek and Roman drama. A covering for the face, to be assumed by each character in the play, its use implied the "outward" appearance or representation of an inner reality. Actors do not wear masks today, yet the *persona* is still retained in our stagecraft through make-up and impersonation of character. Shakespeare's characters are personifications of various human emotions, therefore they wore masks on the stage: Othello, for instance, the mask of jealousy, Macbeth that of ambition, Hamlet that of indecision, Romeo that of love. With masterly insight into the evolution of man he ran the gamut of human character through a succession of masks of men during the voyage from sense to soul. Possibly the immortal bard was not conscious of his great bequest to humanity, but he surely left us a record of our own spiritual history.

We treasure our Shakespeare and the Bible as the two crowning achievements of literary production. In both the process of evolution is markedly similar. In the beginning of his conscious existence man is subject to all external forces and internal passions. His progress is measured by his growth in dominion over these forces and passions. The "Midsummer Night's Dream" of Shakespeare's

youth made man the dupe of imaginary super-
natural spirits. The "Tempest" of his more mature
years gave man, in the guise of *Prospero*, dominion
over creatures of earth and air, wearing the masks
of Caliban and Ariel. In our Bible Adam and Eve
are dupes of evil as symbolized by the serpent;
Jesus vanquished that evil, thus symbolizing the
dominion of man.

But the stage is not the only place where
"masks" are worn. The majority of people off the
stage also meet the world *in persona* or masked.
Charm is often a mask to be assumed or laid aside
at will. Calm suavity may cover a multitude of
irritating fears. The real person behind the mask is
the archetypal being within that unfolds only as
man learns correctly to understand his self. There
is "a spirit in a man." It is manifested in "varieties
of gifts," but it is "the same Spirit," the I AM or
infinite urge set free in the individual self. In each
soul there is a spark of celestial fire, capable of
being fanned into a living flame of manifestation.
No creation of the infinite intelligence can be
purposeless; therefore each human life is important. Otherwise it would not be. Hidden in the
depths of each being is an individual intelligence or
divine personality that is essential to the welfare of
the world, a triumphant personality that gives each

individual his worth or distinction.

What part are you playing in the drama of life? Do you wear a self-hypnotic mask of sickness and failure or do you write your own role from a true conception of the real self within you? Are you expressing that strong, radiant, assertive self which Kant calls the "I knowing"? Do not confuse this with the self-assertiveness of the personal will, which is also a mask—an aping, and imitation—and quite the opposite of that positive state resulting from a knowledge of principle, which is a radiation of an understanding of the divine self.

Astronomers once believed with Ptolemy that the earth was the center around which the sun and the planets revolved. The Copernican system was not promulgated until the sixteenth century. People today are functioning on two levels of consciousness, closely resembling these two astronomical theories. The egotist makes his petty little self the center of his being, assuming that the human self is everything; while the egoist recognizes the ego as that permanent, greater self, that real treasure which is truly his and which cannot be destroyed or stolen from him, that glowing center of his universe from which emanates what we understand to be personality. The earth man is self-centered, grasping, dominant, still under the

"Ptolemaic" spiritual system. The spiritual man has the "sun system" of the universal life and takes his normal position in that life, and this is the "Copernican" system of spiritual adjustment. He has righted himself as regards God and man, reversing the roles of the individual and the universal as completely as Copernicus reversed those of the earth and the sun in astronomical theory.

We all know a solar eclipse to be one of the most superb phenomena that nature offers the human eye. Is it not a potent illustration of the darkness of ignorance, prejudice, and error hiding the real personality? With our discovery of our real personality we emerge from the shadow of all these, just as the sun seems to emerge and shine again when the shadow of the moon has passed. "Believe on the Sun": "Son" or sun, it matters little which way it is written: Son (offspring) of God or sun (center) of self: radiation of Divine Mind! Believe in it! Use it! It is the vital power, the tremendous force, the very center of being.

Because personality is an ultimate reality it is very nearly indefinable. The dictionary calls it "that which constitutes distinction of person; distinctive personal character; individuality." It has been termed "a priceless thing," "the biggest fact in the universe," yet to the average person it suggests only manner or appearance, or tone of voice, or taste in dress. The modern psychologist defines it in terms of physique, temperament, intelligence, instinctive disposition, and the like. Not one and not all of them combined have correctly described the elusive something, the self that made Abraham Lincoln one of the greatest and most powerful personalities every projected across the history of our country.

Homely of face, ungainly of figure, uncouth in dress, what had manner of appearance to do with that mighty American? Why was Plato an outstanding force of his day? What magic did Napoleon use so as to be counted of greater worth than fifty thousand soldiers? What drew multitudes to Phillips Brooks? The casual reader of Walt Whitman is apt to call him an egotist when he reads such lines as "I celebrate myself." When the Nazarene stood in the snyagogue reading from the prophet Isaiah and claiming that He was the fulfillment of that Scripture, many called it blasphemy. We are all familiar with His repeated declaration that He was the son of God. I have heard objections to the line in Gray's "Elegy" that speaks of "mute inglorious Milton" on the ground that a mute Milton is no Milton. Then Romain Rolland writes, "If we had a Boileau, no one would listen

to him." "If they did not listen to him,"
Christophe replied, "he would not be a Boileau."

Shining through the crystal prism of humanity,
God emerges in the component rainbow colors of
great personalities. "Now there are varieties of
gifts, but the same Spirit," the same power, fitted
into each individual mind, to be expressed in each
individual person. Your health is the result of how
much of your real self you are able to manifest.
You have been taught to believe in God. Now learn
about yourself. Believe in what you are, a divine
personality, the ideal of infinite Mind or God.

Our intelligence tells us that man's conception
of deity has evolved as he has grown in wisdom and
knowledge with the advance of civilization. The
universal immanence has gradually developed from
the idea of a God with human characteristics to a
principle of infinity and intelligence beyond any
definition that words or even thought can supply.
God, being eternal, can never change, but man's
understanding of Him cannot be the same as it was
at the dawn of history. A higher order of intelligence reaches for an enlarged ideal, which broadens
with the generations and the centuries as God is
experienced and demonstrated in the lives of men
and women.

We reach God by touching through mind or

spirit what God is: divine personality, infinite Being. Our real personality is what we are expressing of God, that is, what we are in omnipotent Mind. Remember I am not speaking of human personality, which is changeable and unreliable, but of a personality that is an emanation of infinite consciousness. Realization of this personality or self puts us *en rapport* with vast stores of potential energy and touches the hidden spring that releases hitherto unsuspected heights and depths of a personality whose unfailing, illimitable background is God.

Ways of arriving at this understanding are many: metaphysics, science, nature, music, art. No two ways are alike, yet each is a searching for the self in that great storehouse, the mind of God. Your consciousness of yourself is your power of response, not to what you appear to be but what you are potentially. Your true personality depends upon your awareness of your potentialities, your belief in what is actually within you.

Are you aware of these potentialities? Do you respond to your inner possibilities? Forget what you were last year or yesterday. March along and catch up with the spirit of the new era; let go of the old sorrows, old failures, old bodies, old ideas that must inevitably darken your personality. Jesus projected His thought through appearances to the creative source back of them. He dealt with life's problems in the positive assurance that He was one with the Father, dynamic with Divine Mind. You too may come into a newness of life, into a discovery of your dynamic self, and awake in His likeness.

The world today is in a state of material intoxication, of stupefaction from indulgence in the varied cups that materiality offers: cups of money, power, sensuality, of misery, poverty, and death. We must wake up and put away the shadows of unreality, which are but dreams. We must listen to the voice of Him who says, "This is my beloved Son," and take possession of the inheritance of good that has been ours from the beginning.

American soldiers are supplied with numbered identification tags, badges of individuality in relation to a mass or unit. Worn as part of their equipment, the tag is regarded as the ultimate proof of identity; surviving the destruction of outward appearance, it connects the wearer with home and country. Your personality is your tag of identity establishing your relationship to your divine source. It is the distinguishing clue remaining amid the fleeting, warring experiences of sense. It is your undefeatable, victorious "I," offspring of the eternal norm, the prototype of divine personality, the I AM.

Maeterlinck called the human soul "a giant asleep." Surely when it is awakened it must burst its outer coverings of ignorance and fear and become conscious of its original perfection in God's mind. Inevitably it will then cast that "lengthened shadow of a man" which Emerson declared any great accomplishment to be. Many of these giant shadows we have seen projected upon the screen of the world's history. Whatever you achieve is the lengthened shadow of your real personality cast by the "sun" of God, shining through your individual mind and manifesting itself upon your world. Is that shadow wavering and unstable or clearly, truly defined? Is it that of an earth pygmy or that of a heavenly giant?

To be rooted in Divine Mind implies nourishment, life, and growth. Wherever you are, in the home, field, or factory, on the stage, in the studio, or at your desk, God is continually shining through you; He is your substance and your sustenance. He is ever repeating: "I am your servant; use me! In all of your affairs call upon me and I will answer." His answer is your solution to the problem of personality.

You are indeed transformed as you renew your

mind in the correct understanding of personality. You cease conforming to appearances and standards of human belief and hold fast to the divine personality that makes radiant even that which seemed commonplace. As you companion with this presence which clarifies and vivifies, it makes what has been vague definite and renders the negative dynamic. As you strive to perceive this marvelous, eternal idea of true personality, as you work with it in thought, it manifests itself in that magnetic, gracious spirit, in that free, spontaneous expression, the redeemed *persona*.

The Rhythm of Health

The nature lover who has discovered harmony in whistling winds, roaring tempests, raging streams, babbling brooks, and the distant tumult of great cities can appreciate the rapture of the Psalmist when he writes of mountains and hills breaking forth into song and of trees and pastures shouting for joy. Anyone who has lived close to nature understands the underlying rhythm of "the murmuring pines and the hemlocks," the "chime of tinkling rills," winds loosed from their prison repaying "a melody for their liberty received."

Nature's rhythmic quality, that flowing movement which includes all natural phenomena, is evident to all. Silently the tides flood the bays and rivers with a certain regularity in their ebb and flow, twice daily. We hear the song of nature in the murmuring brook, we observe the procession of the seasons, the orderly precision of the appearance and disappearance of light and darkness, of day and night. As the streams of water flow so do streams of that lighter element, air. From the gentle breeze to the fury of the gale, we feel the rhythmic movement of the wind's breath. The very leaves of trees register a rhythmic activity of invisible forces; they grow not in a haphazard manner but arranged in definite patterns of their parent stems.

We live in a world of ceaseless activity, which science terms vibration. Its laws control the transmission of light, heat, and sound. The entire earth literally vibrates with music and is keyed to joyousness. It is not only set to music but is the product of music. Every form of life is rhythmic. All humanity is striving for rhythmical response. Sameness depresses while variety stimulates. Monotony causes physical and mental stupor, while "variety is the spice of life." It swings us into new rhythms. When we swing out of our selfish limitations and feel the pulse of the great whole surging through our being, we may know we are in tune with the infinite One.

We are apt to think of harmony and rhythm in connection only with music, yet the law operates in many other ways, and there are numerous approaches to the rhythm of the universe. As the harmonious, rhythmic expression of life music is everywhere present, recording in our consciousness the wonders of the human body. The inhalation and exhalation of the breath, the diastole and systole of the heart and arteries, establish the rhythmic harmonies of the spiritual world in our mind. As we progress in our study of Truth, we become ever more sensitive to the "music of the spheres." This music continues uninterruptedly, no matter how great the discord may seem to the untrained sense of materiality.

Because every atom of being is thrilling with rhythmic motion, I am convinced that one of the great secrets of health is to be found in harmony and rhythm. The regular movement of life, as seen in action and reaction, is the result of the ceaseless, invisible pulse of the universe. A period of rest and pause inevitably follows stress and action. Rhythm is present in breathing, walking, and swimming. Speech is a result of the pulsing power in lungs and throat.

For the person who finds rhythm and harmony and surrenders himself to them the natural expression is that of freedom, ease, and charm, whether it be expression in speech or song or movement; for the Creator is conscious only of orderly, harmonious existence. He who violates rhythmic order interferes with harmonious action and reaction, thereby cutting himself off from his source of intelligence, energy, and substance. Life and health gradually diminish as we disregard the laws of creation. Our diseases are self-inflicted.

While all motion is rhythmical, various forces cause undulations that vary in rapidity. From the simplest instances of recurring intervals of sound and silence, the primary rhythms, there are generated secondary double, triple, and even quadruple rhythms. But it is not my intention to dwell at length upon the more scientific phase of this subject. I aim simply to reveal the essential points necessary in demonstrating the rhythm of life and health.

The history of mankind discloses that the human race has always instinctively used rhythm as a means of growth and progress. An early Hindu belief was that in the harmony of the spheres was the birthplace of all art and beauty. Ages before the introduction of Christianity Egyptian philosophers pronounced music to be the symbol of the universe, while the ancient Greeks believed musical harmony to be the soul of the cosmos. It was the creed of Pythagoras that all is number and harmony; he based his scientific principles upon the premise that God organized all nature according to the laws of harmony.

In the marvelous Genesis epic of creation we read that the Spirit of creative mind "was moving over the face of the waters," and that God said "Let there be" certain shapes and forms; that light came out of darkness; that the earth was formed out of the void; and that man and natural life appeared where before there had been no living thing. To the student the six days of creation are six periods of evolution, and the entire masterpiece is regarded by him as an allegory. Such a view is necessary to him if he is to keep pace with the truest scientific and philosophic thought, accepting the logical conclusion that it is rhythmic vibration that has shaped plastic substance into tangible form.

Carlyle had rare insight into the subject of creation when he wrote: "See deep enough and you will see musically, the heart of nature being everywhere music, if you can only reach it." Dryden also perceived the idea that "from harmony, from heavenly harmony, this universal frame began." And Emerson, that keen, intelligent observer of life, added his belief that

"The world was built in order

And the atoms marched in tune."

I once saw an experiment by which musical sounds were formed into visible shape. They were produced over a suspended sheet of thin parchment, spread with soft paste, and exquisite forms were shaped out of the plastic medium. Different harmonies produced various shapes of ferns, flowers, and stars. Some form was always developed; never did the paste remain a heterogeneous mass. This tendency of nature is familiar to all who have observed the structure of snowflakes, frost etchings on the windowpane, or the crystallization of minerals. What are all these but music made visible?

As the "world was created by the word of God," so also has the Word been made flesh. As such, it should, according to natural laws, have a beautiful, harmonious, healthy arrangement of form. God, who "commanded the light to shine out of darkness, hath shined in our hearts," and He has given us the power of the Spirit within. It is logical to believe that when we reproduce His notes of exquisite harmony over the suspended parchment of our own subconsciousness, the pliable atoms of our body must be rearranged into forms as harmoniously beautiful as the structures of inanimate nature, much as the pliable substance on the parchment is shaped into beauty by musical sounds.

The power that sustains the natural world also sustains the natural man, although he may but vaguely realize this fact or understand how he can receive the full tide of the illimitable power of countless millions of waves if he will but live in harmony with the rhythmic forces of being. When the rhythm of his being is disturbed through unreasoning emotion or abnormal excitement, invisible ministrants in the realm of radiant energy constantly endeavor to supply him with harmonious conditions. His mind and body seek to restore the usual order and thus prevent exhaustion. Thus the spirit of infinite good is forever radiated in a great, universal wave of harmony, vibrant with life and health.

As man synchronizes his thought with the eternal order of creation, getting in tune with the infinite order, he finds the foundation of health; for to be hale, hearty, and happy one must obey the rhythmic laws of the universe. The wider the range of man's intelligence the greater becomes his use of the universal powers, although his soul rarely becomes aware of the ceaseless vibration, which is energy in motion, as an expression of the one life that is continually manifested in such myriad ways. He seldom recognizes electricity, light, heat, sound, or color as variations of the rhythmic pulse and melodic tendency of universal being.

The term "musical therapy" is of comparatively recent date even though it is not a new idea, having been used by the ancient Greeks. Therapy means cure, and Plato and Pythagoras advocated the use of music for healing, the flute, for instance, for sciatica and the harp for nervous disorders. In his dramatic lyric "Saul," Browning unfolds clearly and succinctly the power of music to restore harmony to a diseased mind. You are doubtless familiar with the Bible story of the incident that inspired the poet's exquisite composition. A brief outline of the poem will suffice to illustrate my idea.

King Saul was suffering from a "mind diseased," and his attendants sent for the boy David, afterward known as both a king and a psalmist. David had previously soothed the monarch with his harp. But now upon entering the king's tent he saw the gigantic figure of Saul, "more black than the blackness," with his arms outstretched on the main pole of the pavilion, hung "drear and stark, blind and dumb."

The young musician tuned up his harp and played first a soothing melody, one that the sheep

knew as they came home to the fold. He followed
this with a martial song. Then he played the help
tune of the reapers and the wine song of their
friendship; then the tender melody of love and
marriage, and the stately religious procession of the
Levites. The tent shook with the shuddering groans
of the king, but his body still hung unmoved.
Again David played, and now he sang:

"Oh, our manhood's prime vigor! No spirit feels
waste,

Not a muscle is stopped in its playing nor sinew
unbraced.

Oh, the wild joys of living!"

Heart, hand, harp, and voice all joined with the
leap of his spirit to lift Saul out of sorrow. "Saul!"
David cried, then stopped and waited to see what
would follow. The king opened his eyes. His dark
hour of death had passed. The harmony of musical
rhythm had brought him back to sanity and life.

The reviving, therapeutic value of music should
be far more generally recognized than it is in this
age of discord. Many physicians who once ridiculed
it are now admitting its value and often prescribing
it as a means of healing. Hospitals and even prisons
are introducing it with good results. Health demands that both mind and body be kept in a state
of harmony. Music affects the emotions, and it is

47

now a well-established fact that the emotions affect the physical functions of glands, heart, and circulation. When moods and emotions are harnessed by scientific understanding, great strides toward health will be made.

Certain harmonious arrangements of ideas in the mind produce like arrangements in the body, quickening the natural functions. In fact, the body is often likened to a highly tuned instrument. We all dread the discordant sounds of an instrument that is out of tune. How carefully the Kreislers and Heifetzes tune their violins before playing. Why? So that they can reproduce the beauty and wonder of rhythm, melody, and harmony. The average person gives much less attention to that most marvelous instrument of all, his body.

It is quite as impossible to produce harmony in the body by drawing upon all nervous and muscular force at one time as it is to get music from jangling all the keys of a piano at once. Each chord and note in its right place and at its proper time, produces a glory of harmony. Likewise the secret of living rhythmically lies in knowing how to regulate the body so that some part of the organism is always at rest while another part is functioning. For rhythmical action is nature's law and must be obeyed if one would live harmoniously.

Every person who perceives the therapeutic value of harmony enlarges his racial consciousness with regard to the healing power of rhythm. Who can say what he may be able to accomplish when all his forces are brought into play and he knows how properly to harmonize and control them! Daily the idea is advancing that there is a tonic property in music that stimulates and re-energizes as well as soothing and relaxing patients. In hospital work it has been found to produce not only emotional diversion but results of lasting benefit. Personally I have known it to banish a severe headache, to assuage a burning fever, and to restore sight and speech lost through shell shock.

To be mentally harmonious is to have a body correctly attuned to life and health. Daily scientific thinking is the only means that will attune man to harmonious conditions. No musician would tune his instrument one day and then forget to do so for a week. Yet we are just as negligent as that as regards our individual attunement or adjustment. In Plato's "Republic" there is a passage that says:

"To him that has an eye to see there can be no fairer spectacle than that of a man who combines the possession of moral beauty in his soul with outward beauty of form, corresponding and harmonizing with the former, because the same great pattern enters into both. My belief is that a good body will, not by its own excellence make the soul good, but on the contrary, that a good soul will, by its excellence, render the body as perfect as it can be."

Every thought is rhythmic if it accords with universal or spiritual harmonies. Nature is alive with vibration, rhythm, and harmony. The individual who aligns himself with nature's constructive principle must be restored to health and happiness. In his "Dance of Life" Havelock Ellis says: "The diversity of the many is balanced by the stability of the one. That is why life must always be a dance, for that is what a dance is: perpetual, slightly varied movements which are always held true to the shape of the whole."

He continues with the thought that not only life but the universe is a dance; for the universe is made up of a certain number of elements—less than a hundred—and the "periodic law" of these elements is metrical. A wonderful unison is exhibited in the dance, the mass moving as "a single being, stirred by a single impulse." Industrial and social unification would result from the same idea being applied to practical affairs.

Christianity is both the religion and the science of harmony. The teaching of the Master was very definite on the point of the heavenly harmony that is creation. It is strange that we have lost the true significance of the word heaven, upon the idea of which Jesus dwelt so insistently. We have made it a place although it has no reference to place. It is a condition of mind: that of harmony.

The Master taught men how to be in harmony with the universe and practice rhythmic living. Have you ever paused to wonder why Jesus said that all things would be added? He knew the law of demonstration, namely that if a person seeks and finds the realm of harmony, he will naturally be supplied with every needed thing: life, health, abundance. All good comes to those who are harmonious. To prove what the Master proved we must first strike the chord of Christianity: rhythm, harmony, heaven.

The Manifestation of Health

If you would master the science of spiritual healing, you must understand the law of manifestation. By manifestation I mean a movement outward, a bodying forth of something, a result of some cause. I am sure every rational person acknowledges the material world as a world of phenomena or appearances: a reflection or expression of something. Such a person will also admit that there cannot be a shadow without the substance of something behind it. For everything of which we see the symbol there is the reality, preexistent and substantial.

When you come to see that the truly existing things are ideas, you understand that the actually existent world is the spiritual or mental. Every tangible effect then becomes a product of some quality of consciousness, an expression of a force back of its material manifestation. To spiritual vision the entire universe is soul substance in expression, embodiment of living intelligence, the "Word . . . made flesh" in a variety of celestial castings. The visible body has an invisible background, the material circumstance has an intangible setting, the practical development has a spiritual agent. All objectified form once existed only in the subjective realm.

If material things are dependent upon ideas and the natural world is but the human way of perceiving immortal entities, we then recognize mind as the reality back of that which appears as the body. We might say that the body is formulated Spirit, for man is a manifestation of divine Principle; through him as the epitome of Being the omnipotent Spirit is expressed.

The seer of Genesis saw clearly that "God made the earth . . . and [every] herb of the field" in the heavens, before the material form was expressed. We are told in this allegorical story of creation that "the Spirit of God was moving" and manifestation resulted. Principle expressed itself in form. Until this fundamental law of creation is understood, there can be no intelligent progress in spiritual science.

In studying the process of manifestation we learn that the first movement in the mind of God was pure thought; movement commensurate with the active force of thought is necessarily projected in some form of expression. Pure thought controls the inorganic universe and supervises the active force whose misdirection could so easily work annihilation. But the work of Divine Mind is exact and dependable. Atoms and molecules respond to it. Grapes are not manifested from thorns, nor figs from thistles. Planets neither crash nor collide. Yet man is disorderly and inharmonious.

If it is an absolute law of being that man and his world are representations of what he has seen with his mind, where there is no mental type there will be no material form. Visual perception is casual, and when the mind does not see there is no material effect. The sight of which I am speaking does not come through the vision of externals, nor is it dependent upon optical organs. A Hindu metaphysician throws a ray of light on the subject: "Thou canst not behold Me with thy two outer eyes. I have given thee an eye divine."

Seeing nothing but the ideas in our own mind, we are bound within the material walls of our own misconceptions as long as the models in our consciousness are "of the earth, earthy." The "eye divine" is the organ of spiritual insight into the body. When the mind disagrees with a belief, it causes what Paul called "discord in the body." The true idea of body is "cosmic vision" or the agreement of the mind with itself.

According to some metaphysicians, we see through our organism in one, two, and three dimensions. The fourth dimension is attained by those who earnestly seek spiritual discernment or who are receptive to the ideas of pure reason. This dimension is an evolution out of human consciousness, the three-dimensional consciousness, into a spiritual kingdom.

Cosmic vision is the spiritual aspiration that brings into being the new organism or body, enabling us to "see" in four dimensions. If the body is not healed, there has been no conception of the true body, which cannot think or act on the basis of old, imperfect beliefs. There is a way out of the reactions of the subconscious, and that is by the science of Christ.

Christianity reveals the ideal body, the model that must be held in consciousness. As we hold fast to this revelation of the divine model we shall be transformed into it. This real or perfect body is man's gift from his Father; it cannot be taken away from him or injured in any way. Jesus demonstrated His power over what we call the material body through His perception of the glorified body, "eternal in the heavens," that we must claim as our original body.

Man's true mission is to be a cocreator with God, an interpreter of pure intelligence, a supervisor of the work of living molecules, an architect of cosmic design. All material has been furnished him; innately he holds the magic formula of perfect manifestation. His mind is the dwelling place of the thought activity that should operate in accord with and coordinate with the infinite purpose. His mind or spirit is his point of contact with his Father source; for competent direction of his thought he may have the "mind of Christ."

If a man would think truly—according to Principle—always basing his thought upon the divine idea, his manifestations would be perfect and his body would function ideally. But he has erected a barrier of sensation between himself and the source of his being, and these sense manifestations so attract him that he loses sight of his spiritual ideal and thus cuts himself off from the Fountainhead.

Life in its manifestation requires law for its protection and growth, but many do not see that law is the basis of spiritual demonstration as surely as it is of natural phenomena. They do not recognize the fact that orderly method relates and connects events, not accidentally or by chance but surely and definitely, not sometimes but at all times, not in certain places but everywhere, not for special people but for humanity.

A manifestation of spiritual healing is a miracle to one who has not seen or experienced it and does not understand its principles. But to many it is not an unusual event but a result of understanding and of compliance with law. There is a perfect plan that presupposes, at least potentially, an expression free from imperfection. If such a manifestation is possible, there is a way to attain it. If there is a way, surely all must be seeking it.

Life exists in every cell and organ of the body, waiting to be stirred into activity. Its stimulation requires no miraculous power. It is always there, the strongest force in the universe, ready to respond. God creates in the ideal; man carries out what God has idealized. But man must first have a vision of the ideal, and it does not abide with those who are willing to bend every effort toward working out its fulfillment. Persistent action must back it up; otherwise it is not a vital conviction.

When we understand the "real body" and our responsibility as regards its manifestation, we realize that it is entitled to our most exacting courtesy and consideration. We know that the author in preparing his manuscript, the artist in painting his picture, the sculptor in shaping his clay thus expresses his inner vision and reveals his spiritual ideal. None of these would think of neglecting his finished product, allowing it to be mutilated or defaced, to become worn and faded from lack of appreciative care. Each values, protects, and cherishes his work as the concrete embodiment of his ideal. The more perfect it is the more persistently he guards it from injury and seeks to retain its original perfection of expression.

A God who rules through law is far more dependable than one who can be influenced and changed by man's cries of discontent. Intelligence recognizes Him as everliving, ever active, and ever present in His creation, as self-existent principle, filling the universe and surrounding us on every side with manifestations of His creative activity, always at work in compliance with orderly law.

There are definite laws governing the care and use of the body, and it is each person's duty to employ these in maintaining the rhythmic order of nature in the functioning of the various parts of the organism, whose harmonious coordination is necessary to that effortless action which is the manifestation of health, the true expression of the "real body."

Nature has provided ways and means for protecting and sustaining physical health. The life force should sweep through the body in a torrent of cleansing, purifying, vitalizing activity. Every one of nature's provisions for preserving a sound, whole organism should be encouraged. Life-giving methods should be persistently practiced. Forces of nature, so ready to cooperate in establishing a healthy organism, must be utilized.

The body is wonderfully constructed, having within it the power to perform all functions necessary to its operative activity. Every cell is intelligent and capable of renewing itself. In its chemical laboratory it separates and combines, selects and rejects component elements and sends them on their mission of nutrition. Its involuntary action and reaction employ the "breath of the Almighty" in its life-sustaining function.

As long as man through conscious mental control exerts his intelligence in keeping a normal, harmonious balance among its requirements, the body cannot disintegrate. Only neglect or misdirected energy produces disturbance and destruction. Its remarkable composition requires perfect adjustment of each organ and function to all others. It is a great unity, and its equilibrium must be preserved. The way to be well is to be whole, and wholeness implies having all the original parts in harmonious relation, in perfect order.

In addition to exercise, deep breathing, food, recreation, and sleep, the rebuilding tissue used up in daily work demands spiritual understanding of Divine Mind; for it has been proved by scientific experiment how persistently the mental state affects the process of cell activity in the body. Mind is the creative force back of physical well-being. Desire, resolute purpose, and enthusiastic, steadfast effort are required in the manifestation and maintenance of bodily health.

Keeping the natural laws instituted by the Creator is the working principle of manifestation. To believe blindly that some mysterious power outside the body is going to descend upon and vitalize it, or to ask God to heal something we have brought upon ourselves by disobeying His orderly laws, is not only futile but unintelligent. Within itself there is sufficient power to heal and restore the body. If we are too inert to study and use and direct what is already ours, we cannot expect a perfect manifestation of health.

"Is any one among you suffering? Let him pray." These are words of the apostle James, who adds that the fervent, earnest prayer of a righteous man avails much, but he goes on to explain that clear understanding of the relation between the idea and its fulfillment is necessary. "Faith apart from works is dead." To beseech God to come and heal our diseases when we will not exert ourselves to keep His laws is unreasonable and unproductive.

I would not have you understand that life-giving methods relate principally to the rules of hygiene and sanitation, to the preservation of physical health. I would have you recognize something much more profound: the law *back* of diet, fresh air, and pure water for the body. I believe in making use of every one of nature's provisions for sustaining and renewing physical life and keeping the living organism sound and whole. However the more we learn about the body and the orderly intelligence at work in each individual cell the better we comprehend the possibilities of mind control. As we note the chemical effect produced in the body by varying states of consciousness, we must conclude that the mental state is far more important than it has been regarded to be and that it has a therapeutic function that cannot be disputed.

We exist as the atoms composing God's great universe, much as the atoms of our body make up our individual entity. We are related to our atoms as God is related to us as human beings. Disorder exists in our human universe because individuals refuse to recognize their relationship to God and to each other. Disorder exists in our body also because of lack of coordination, but with this difference: man has the free will to choose his course of action. His atoms have not; they are dependent upon his direction. If through well-directed, intelligent thought man reinforces their natural tendency toward wholeness, they automatically respond to the order he establishes for their activity. Through thought the intelligence of order or the disruptive effect of disorder sweeps through man's individual universe and is manifested in harmony or discord.

Our intelligence is a part of God's consciousness. We have received it in order that we may understand the mystic laws of harmony and coordination that we are expected to obey. As we allow His life and intelligence to flow through us, by means of thought they pervade each cell and tend always to restore it to its original state of divine order.

Thus God weaves and reweaves Himself into the immortal cells of our body, and with the warp and woof of mind, these cells, individually perfect, are woven into and manifested in the many organs of our body. Thus divine grace is inherent in each cell and each organ receives potentially the possibility of perfect functioning.

In our body these cells are continually being renewed; they are plastic, moldable cells. In our mind images are eternally taking shape. Cellular activity is not dependent upon us, but cellular form is our responsibility and depends upon the images we hold in mind. True ideas are transmitted to us from divine intelligence, but they can reach us as such only through a pure and unobstructed medium. Until we learn to control our human, negative beliefs and opinions they will continue to distort our manifestations of well-being.

Through his higher understanding man will come to realize that for him to despise, neglect, or debase his body is to dim the divine spark within him and to dishonor the source of his being. But when he regards his body as a temple that houses the "essence of life," he builds after the image and likeness of his Creator.

Daily we are contacting yesterday's thought manifestations, even while we are forming patterns for those of tomorrow. As we comprehend and work with Principle we find within ourself the power to manifest perfect conditions in our body, to form and transform it according to the living image we hold in mind.

Restoring the Soul

Whenever I speak of restoring the soul my thought inevitably reverts to the 23d Psalm and its message of calm, quiet trust. Its series of terse, vivid expressions are strung like fine-cut cameos on a wire of faith: faith in and dependence upon a power higher than my own. The Psalmist wrote straight from a heart illumined by the serene tranquillity of absolute trust in the intelligent guidance, the tender protection, and the ample provision of that power.

A clearer realization of the beauty of the Psalms came to me when I saw the deep ravines and overtowering mountains of Palestine. I could easily imagine them infested with wild beasts and robbers lying in wait, and the often repeated symbolism of sheep and shepherd, in the Bible, became peculiarly appropriate to my mind. It was then that the

"Shepherd Psalm," as it has been called, illuminated my consciousness with its exquisite beauty of illustration: green pastures and still waters and a shepherd's tender care.

The beauty of the Psalms lies in their quick change from material to spiritual terms. "He restores my soul" instantly transports us from the refreshment of water and food and protection to reinvigoration of spirit. Just as a good shepherd sees that the sheep are fed and watered, guarded and guided, so the Good Shepherd leads and cares for us, protecting us through the dark watches of the night of trouble, restoring our soul, and leading us in right paths "for his name's sake."

We see many unhappy faces, faces sullen and rebellious, emaciated by want and suffering, or bearing the marks of surfeit and dissipation. Where are men to find the strong moral courage to reconstruct and rebuild their life? Where except in a restoration of soul? When the rain falls and the flood rises, there is a safe fold where all may find shelter under the watchful eye of the shepherd. The varied experiences of life are material in the sense that they involve material means. But it is the spiritual that must come first in any misfortune. The Lord is our shepherd, and it is to Him we must turn for that inner refreshment which is the soul's restoration.

Health of soul furnishes the fundamental life-giving state that produces physical soundness. The healthy soul radiates its thought force to the physical body. Thought is the electric connection between mind and matter, providing the means of contact with the soul, or source of power. Thought adjusting itself to the perfect vibration of infinite life results in health. Failing to harmonize with the divine order of Being, it produces the jangling static of nonadjustment and failure.

Discordant emotions disturb the forces of the soul and are pictured forth in the body as disease or disorder. They change the chemical action of the blood and vital fluids, creating a poison that vitiates the life stream. True scientific healing is an operation of the inner life force, working through mind and thought, outward, from the origin or cause back of the body effect.

Drugs do not affect emotions of the soul, neither do they heal the physical consequence of indulgence in harmful emotions, although they have been used for many years in treating the effects of erroneous thought on the body. As an expression of infinite life man is a unit, not a conglomeration of functioning organs. Any interruption of the natural flow of life causes suffering to all members of the body. The intelligent treatment recognizes this lack of isolation or detachment in the physical organism, knowing that in every part the whole is implied, and that spiritual healing depends upon a consciousness of constant contact with the universal soul of Being. The way to be well is to be whole; and wholeness implies having all the essential or original parts in harmonious relationship, complete, entire, and in perfect order.

We are fortunate to have a standard of perfection whereby to model our life; to have the privilege of accepting the great Master's sweeping invitation to find inward calmness and rest. Jesus, world teacher, knew the sorrows and griefs of humanity. He was a master of the art of living. He was especially interested in human nature and the barriers it sets up against its divine sonship. We may learn from Him, if we will, about the roots of hidden tension, the strain that we find at times almost unbearable.

Most people have hidden germs of unhappiness and failure locked up in their memories. They are usually amazed to be told that these are secret infections which poison the mind and spirit and are intimately connected with ill-health, unhappiness, and business difficulties. Mental tension weakens the efficiency and vigor, and relief can be found only by searching the heart for lurking enemies and crowding them out of consciousness, thus restoring the soul to its original state of harmony.

The word *tension* calls to mind something pulled or stretched to its very breaking point. Whatever it happens to be, whether thread or rope, sinew or nerve filament, a condition or a relationship, it indicates stress or strain to an extreme degree. A tight thread destroys the uniformity of a stitch and spoils the seam or the web of which it is a part. A strained sinew causes disorder in the muscular tissue of the body. A tense nerve filament carries warped impulses to its central power station, the brain.

Relaxation is a release from strain, a loosening of tension. It opens the door to an inner renewal; it restores the soul. All force is rhythmic and travels in waves, rising and falling, advancing and retreating. For every wave, there is a crest and a calm. This principle of undulation is one of the fundamental laws of the body. Even the heart action, which many believe to be continuous, includes a brief instant of rest after each beat. In this fraction of a second it gains renewed vigor for its next effort. Nerve and thought force move in the same manner if we allow them to do so.

When wave activity becomes that of flood or deluge, it results in destruction. To keep the mental forces going in a continuous flood of energy is to inundate and weaken them. It is working against law and reduces the efficiency of our efforts. The ability to shift the burden of care and anxicty for a brief period of rest is the secret of tremendous energy.

Instead of toiling to get more knowledge, happiness, or substance, we need that tranquillity of soul which can "be still, and know" what we already have that is of real value. Life has something to tell each one of us, but it cannot be heard above the turmoil of hurry or the jangle of jealous resentment; the discord of yesterday's disappointment or the clamor of tomorrow's pessimism. We need to pause and find a still, strong power behind the mysterious process of growth. To respond thus is not to be sluggish or inactive. It is nature's formula for expansion; it is quiet calm poised at the center of vital activity.

Every person owes it to himself to find this secret, silent place to which he may "fly away, and be at rest" from human associations that weary him because of their inharmony; this place where he may find a sense of freedom from the adverse conditions and diverse tasks to which he feels the need of constant readjustment, and find relaxation and restoration of soul.

No person can give of himself, of his high thoughts and impulses, before he is, in a sense, free from "personalities." Only in the quiet of his own being can he discover his potentialities and develop a clear, wholesome consciousness of his real self. Only here can he work out his problems, measure his capabilities, and find his true work. When he thus enters into the inner chamber and shuts the door he is contemplating the Father as the source of all his good. In his approach to the "secret place of the Most High" he identifies himself with the universal intelligence and finds that "peace of God, which passes all [human] understanding."

Peace and power are inherent gifts that we may all possess. No person is truly great until he has attained the harmony of spirit that is found at the true axis of his being, the place of absolute stillness within the soul, where the peace of God reigns and where tumultuous race thought and sensuous belief cannot reach.

"Let not your hearts be troubled, neither let them be afraid." It is the Master's farewell message to His friends. "Peace I leave with you; my peace I give to you." His was a peace of soul that nothing could disturb; a peace that remained serene in the midst of cruel betrayal, unjust accusation, and atrocious punishment.

The Master, living in constant contact with the universal source of vitality, issued a great invitation, including the major portion of the human race: "Come to me, all who labor and are heavy laden, and I will give you [the secret of] rest." Surely the worth of His achievements establishes the authority of His assurance: "Learn from me . . . and you will find rest for your souls."

In our recognition of the interdependence of body, mind, and spirit, we need to realize and to practice a relaxation of tenseness in all three. Well do we know its reactive effect upon the mental and the physical. How are we going to apply it to the spiritual? "Learn from me . . . and you will find rest for your souls." What was the secret of that inner repose which faced disappointment and betrayal, reviling and injustice, weariness and death with the dignity and majesty of quiet calm?

"Come unto me, and I will give you rest." It is the Teacher's invitation: "Come"—not to His personality but to His consciousness of well-being, His divine insight into Truth. In this quietness and confidence you shall find strength to live as He did; to be uplifted as He was; to enter, as He did, the very kingdom of heaven on earth.

The Yoke of Yesterdays

"Behold, I create new heavens and a new earth; and the former things shall not be remembered." "If any one is in Christ, he is a new creation, the old has passed away." These are the words of Isaiah and Paul throwing off the yoke of yesterdays, which is a barrier to progress. More recently we have listened to Walt Whitman renouncing the corpse of his old self, which he had cast off and left behind him; and we have hailed Tennyson immortalizing the idea of rising on stepping-stones of his dead self to higher things.

There are so many heirs to the slavery of the old yesterdays constantly looking backward toward things that should long since have been blotted out and forgotten. Whatever the success that attended past methods, new conditions of life demand new attitudes and improved ways. Fixed ideas develop into mental habits, and it becomes difficult to adjust the mind to changed circumstances and different environments. But these will not change by shaping themselves to us; it is we who must make the necessary adjustments. It is imperative that the consciousness should be free of the bondage and limitations to which past prejudices and traditions have subjected it. Superstition, creed, dogma, doubt, fear—all are bars to freedom.

Jesus used the word *repent* in the sense of taking a new attitude. "Repent, for the kingdom of heaven is at hand." What this kingdom has in store for you depends upon your flexibility of mind and your willingness to readjust your ideas and beliefs to its requirements. It is a natural human impulse to feel that conditions should be adjusted by changes made on the outside, by changes in anything but the inner self.

But adjustment is a mental course of action. The divine law of adjustment, when understood and practiced, corrects and regulates every disorder in human experience. When the outer individual self is adjusted to the inner spiritual self, belief in the power of objective conditions is surmounted and all barriers are broken down.

There is a spiritual significance back of all material appearance. Living in an inharmonious atmosphere is unnecessary, because the law of mental adjustment is the same law that operates in tangible manifestation. If you find you cannot adjust yourself to outside conditions you may know that your consciousness is not harmoniously adjusted in spirit. The divine law of adjustment contains a principle by which all discord, confusion, and inharmony is corrected and regulated. It transports the consciousness to a higher plane where all relationships are perfectly maintained. It recognizes one law, the law of good, which is the law of all life.

Paul preached with zealous energy the gospel of putting away the old and being renewed or readjusted in the spirit of the mind. He included the release of all bitterness and anger, all malice and evil-speaking, and with great fervency he declared his purpose of forgetting the past and reaching forward to the future, of pressing on toward his goal. He said, "I die every day." Each night was a sleep and a forgetting, each morning a renewal and a transformation.

Is there something in your storehouse of memory over which you are secretly brooding? Some unhappy recollection that terrifies you with its constant recurrence? Some hidden bitterness or hatred that nourishes a burning desire to even up an old score? Some sense of resentment against injustice? We have all experienced the destructive agency of such unbridled emotion; we know the indigestion that results from anxiety, the headache that has its source in angry irritation or depressed discouragement. We have observed the workings of protracted grief, cherished resentment, or bitter envy in many a case of chronic invalidism.

In reading of the healings of Jesus it seems as though His entire system of therapeutics rested upon the one word *forgiveness.* "Which is easier to say . . . 'Your sins are forgiven,' or to say, 'Rise . . . and walk'?" He knew the remedy for those weary and heavy-laden ones, the secret of freedom from the tension that was holding them in physical bondage. His magic word was *forgiveness.* He sometimes called it *nonresistance.* That old law of an eye for an eye had accomplished little in their lives.

Revenge, requital, and retribution do not liberate the troubled mind. Jesus knew and practiced a more excellent way. He likened the old method to cleansing the outside of a cup or platter and allowing the inside to remain soiled from past use, thus producing contamination that could be counteracted only by removing the cause. Setting the heart or inner man to rights would expel misery from the outer.

"A man who foolishly does me wrong—I will return to him the protection of my ungrudging love: the more evil that comes from him the more good shall come from me. Hatred does not cease by hatred at any time; hatred ceases by love. This is an old rule," Buddha wrote. Surely this was the rule Jesus taught and lived: forgiveness. He recognized it as a complete formula for liberation from the tense habits that produce many physical ills. "Repay no one evil for evil" was Paul's interpretation of the Christ consciousness. "Live peaceably with all. . . . Be not overcome by evil, but overcome [give over] evil with [for] good."

Forgiveness is a liberator born of love and springing from the "hidden man of the heart." It means to give something for or on account of something else. It includes much more than overlooking an injury. An even exchange must be arranged: justice for injustice, good for evil, praise for criticism, love for hate. As you give so shall you receive. It is the law of compensation resting upon a basis of immutable principle.

Forgiving is "giving for" and placing in the consciousness a realization of freedom from something that causes pain or disturbs our ease. Sin is missing the mark, because we fail to perceive and apply spiritual principles. According to the old belief, sin was an infraction of social ethics, but we now know that it is far more inclusive. It is every thought and act that does not measure up to spiritual reality. Its manifestations are appalling, because it is the nature of thought to become visible.

The old teaching that God forgives sin only when we beseech Him is not in accordance with Truth. Sin and evil cannot be separated from their consequences; they are as intimately related as the root and the branch. They are the result of thinking outside of principle, thereby failing to measure up to the absolute. Forgiveness of sin is the Biblical term for changing our misconception of life for the truth, and we do this in direct ratio to our perception of the true reality.

The new thought of Christianity is that man, not God, forgives sin. That it is but the false concept of life that leads us to sin will of course sound revolutionary to many, who will not understand that when we perceive reality we correct the errors of sense in our own mind and that of others. But we know that God holds man eternally in the perfection of spirit, and as infinite Mind can never be influenced by the error that blinds man to the ideal vision of himself, it can never change its concept of the Divine Son. However, before this concept is established in the human consciousness, its opposing belief must be eliminated. As we correct our mistaken ideas we forgive our own sins, by "giving" our belief in evil "for" a knowledge of truth.

Because Jesus saw so clearly the spiritual reality of man as an ideal image and because He could discriminate between evil and the perfection sustained in God thought, He had the ability to "take away" or "forgive" the sins of the world. We too may follow His example and forgive the sins of the race if we will refuse to judge by the appearance and exercise "righteous judgment" instead. To do this it is necessary to recognize man as an infinite idea of infinite Mind and to refuse to stamp upon the consciousness as real the mistakes that have been made.

"If you forgive the sins of any, they are forgiven; if you retain the sins of any, they are retained." Thus the Christian religion defines our responsibility. Every forward step in the evolution of humanity is taken by correcting error in the race thought. To "heal the sick, raise the dead, cleanse lepers, cast out demons" is the natural result of the forgiveness of sin; wholeness automatically results when evil beliefs are cast out. If you are a Christian student, you must hold the real consciously in your vision, and each person who does this helps to set the world free from its delusion of the power of material misconceptions. Sustained in thought, belief in evil as existent makes it an active force; so it appears to be all the imagination has made it.

"Repent, and believe in the gospel" is the admonition of the great Teacher in urging a remission of sin through change of thought, through belief in the "good news" that the Father has never been an angry God dealing out punishment for sin. In the new thought of Christianity repentance is a form of denial, and forgiveness of sin is an erasure from the consciousness of a material misconception.

As an illustration we have Jesus' word picture of the prodigal son arrogantly and rebelliously leaving the protecting plenty of his father's house, only to return ashamed and humiliated, expecting to be punished by disinheritance and debasement. A true symbol this, not of the Father's angry imprecations but of His constant, expectant watchfulness for the return of a son—never a thought of punishment or reproach, but an advance to meet the loved one, to heap honors upon him, and to restore him to a sonship that had never even been questioned. It was a cause for merrymaking too, because "your brother was dead, and is alive; he was lost and is found."

So he told them this parable as another picture of repentance. This time Jesus symbolized the loving yearning of the Father by the tenderness of a shepherd whose watchful care follows the lost sheep into the terrors of darkness, rescuing and restoring him to the peaceful safety of the fold, and there is more joy at the finding of the one that is lost than there is over the ninety-nine that remain always safe.

I am sure you could not interpret these illustrations as an encouragement to sin or to refuse to repent. In both instances sufficient punishment was suffered as a direct result of error, for sin and its consequences are always united. Jesus never recognized or emphasized repentance as the old law taught it; He preferred to dwell upon the good or "righteous" rather than upon the evil. His healings were pure demonstrations of the forgiveness of wrong thinking and its consequent results. We are beginning to understand that when He forgave sin it meant to Him a release from the heavy yoke of yesterdays, a change of thought, a healing of the mind; and the natural result of all this was freedom and restoration of the body.

"Thou preparest a table before me in the presence of mine enemies." We may not be sure of the meaning the Psalmist intended, but we know what Jesus' interpretation would have been. He knew that a man's enemies are not human beings but his own error thoughts: his belief in lack, in sickness and death, his worries, fears, and anxieties. Against these alien enemies, these beliefs in physical, mental, and financial imperfection, our human efforts seem weak and fragile. Right "in the presence" of these enemies a table of plenty is prepared, where each is an honored guest: "Thou anointest my head with oil." Each one's "cup runneth over" with health, life, and substance.

We must learn to turn away from fighting against conditions by "forgiving" them, by letting the brilliant rays of truth banish their shadowy darkness. Then flooding ideas of health and wholeness will crowd out and expunge from the subconscious mind the morbid beliefs of sickness and disease. Forgiveness goes hand in hand with forgetfulness; for when one is not willing to forget, how is one able to forgive? Forgiveness is only perfected by forgetfulness; by letting "the dead past bury its dead."

We must forgive and forget as we would that our own errors should be forgiven and forgotten by others. "Forgive us our debts, as we also have forgiven our debtors" is the prayer Jesus taught His disciples. It should teach us the futility of resenting trifling injuries, of wishing to "get even" with those who criticize or ridicule us. The Master's reaction to bitter injustice was "Father, forgive them."

To forgive *as* we would be forgiven is the very crux of our mental need. Forgiveness is essentially a function of the mind. It clears the channel through which Divine Mind flows into its individual outlets. Always remember this. To forgive is to remit, to absolve, to set free from the bondage of yesterday's yoke, to give something for something. The channel through which your forgiveness flows to another is the same channel through which the forgiveness of others flows to you. If you obstruct its flow by denying it to your fellow men, you raise a barrier between yourself and God. As you would be forgiven, so you must forgive.

I am often surprised to find so little understanding in persons who earnestly desire to be healed of sickness and poverty. They hold locked in their memories the buried microbes of dormant ailments, injurious to the mind and closely associated with their lack of health and supply. I find such people secretly brooding over past injury or injustice, resenting criticism and unkindness, or reproaching themselves for mistakes.

Before there can be any outward expression of healing I am sure it is positively necessary to heal the havoc that bitterness and ill will create in the human mind. Perhaps it is, as many declare, humanly impossible to forget or forgive such wrongs as some have experienced. The human nature cannot accomplish this. It is the divine nature that extends mercy, love, and pardon. From your human standpoint it is difficult, often seemingly impossible, to condone an offense. Yet surely there was nothing of human nature in that prayer from the Cross: "Father, forgive them; for they know not what they do."

Forgiveness erases inharmony, anger, and jealousy, searching back of the petty faults and trivial mistakes of humanity until it beholds the true spiritual or Christ man. It indicates a removal of erroneous conceptions, a "giving them over" for a like measure of freedom and peace of spirit. As it corrects mistakes it cancels beliefs in evil and records only knowledge of truth. It springs from your soul, the innermost part of you. It is not genuine unless it totally erases every memory of bitterness. Its vision is broad; it sees beyond the petty faults of human nature to the actual spiritual self that is shining behind the clouds of limitation. It discovers the "Divine Son" in every individual.

You may be surprised to hear that first of all you must forgive yourself. If you are torturing your mind with thoughts of retribution for sins and shortcomings, you will remain bound until you make remission of your own faults by realizing the forgiving love of the indwelling Father, who grants you the power to free yourself and others. When you have given your thoughts of discontent, resentment, faultfinding, hate, and lack for their mental opposites, the conditions of your life and your affairs are going to undergo a radical change.

Forgive your brother, yourself, your "fate," if that is what you call it. Forgive everything and everybody. Forgive, not once but even "seventy times seven." It is the only way to drop the yoke of yesterdays and remove the obstruction between yourself and freedom. Forgive and forget those things that lie in your past. Blot out of your memory the misery of your unhappy experiences. Demolish the old structures of worthless retrospection. Let the "first things" pass away, and behold, "all things" shall be made new in your life. Give up your hatreds and criticism for love and praise; your selfish gloom for joyous radiations of confident expectancy; your suspicion and distrust for faith in eternal goodness. Each one of these substitutes will accomplish rich results in your life.

"According to Your Faith"

What did Jesus mean when He said, "According to your faith be it done to you"? Faith in what? He Himself answered the question: "Have faith in God." We take this to mean faith in a power greater than the human self and close relations with this power; an ability to draw upon and appropriate its principles in the absolute conviction that it will respond to our demand. The world is alive and immortal as man is alive and immortal. All things that compose the earth are eternal ideas in the radiant consciousness of God, and faith enables us to so discern them. Faith is the purity through which we see God's face; without it we walk in darkness.

Jesus found men anxiously seeking relief from their ills in material remedies, but as these cannot reach mental causes they fall short of effecting the desired healing. It was the way the Master saw life that enabled Him to heal effectively, for true healing is agreement with God, and only faith gives the ability to agree with the eternal goodness that is God. Faith is enlarged vision, true insight into life. Jesus' vision was so keen that He perceived at once the false sense under which men labored and the mental pitfalls into which they fell because of this. His sympathy went out to them, as ours does to those who are physically blind, and He spent His life endeavoring to correct their spiritual blindness by inducing His own faith into their consciousness.

The Master saw fear as a prolific cause of disease, because in this disturbed state a person's mind cannot be receptive to the faith that accomplishes healing; therefore many times His injunction was "Fear not!" He well knew that fear is a parasite living upon other emotions and absorbing their very life substance. Today we recognize it as each man's enemy, which he is called upon to face single-handed. It causes more havoc in the human system than any other emotion or condition, yet it is irrational and absurd. Absolutely without foundation, it produces utter chaos. It is a poor negative but the instigator of countless positives. It is Hydra-headed, and its annihilation is a Herculean task until one knows how to apply the firebrand of faith after each decapitation. We must either master fear or it will master us, as it invariably finds expression in the body and exerts a paralyzing effect upon the organism.

Faith, which is the "substance" of all good, must pierce through the fear shadows to that which really is. Seeing with the enlightened eyes of faith, we can maintain a transcendent, definite attitude of thought. We know that our body exists because the idea or soul of it is in infinite Mind. To perceive this soul is to gain dominion over it, and this dominion is a state of faith. We all possess this faculty of faith perception, and to keep perpetually functioning in conscious contact with our spiritual source should be the high endeavor of our life. We may keep this sustained contact with the spiritual world through a .correct exercise of our perceptive faculties.

The self-conscious mind of humanity is negative as a result of dimness of vision. To see positively we must have spiritual illumination. We must receive the same mind "which was also in Christ Jesus." But in our modern world most of us are so actively engaged in *getting* health, or whatever it is we are pursuing, that we fail to pause long enough to receive the quickening power. We need to cultivate the deep tranquillity of soul that can "be still, and know." Healing must be approached in the receptive attitude that listens for the "still small voice," which cannot be heard above the turmoil and discord of hurried activities but is dependent upon the passive receptivity, the quiet calm, at the center of our being. In the secret place of the soul we replenish our strength by turning the passive self toward the intelligible world and receiving the inner word from the healing silence.

Too often we overestimate the value of dynamic force, losing sight of the receptive quality; the passive is ignored in the rush of active principle. We fret and hurry to accomplish our healing through continuous, laborious effort, searching restlessly in the outer for something that must be discovered within. We forget that the human mind is made up of two elemental principles: one is the intellectual or active; the other the receptive or passive. A conjunction of thought and feeling, of idea and sensation, is required to form a concrete reality. In all nature's creative process there is activity, passivity, and form; the urge or essence, the neutral or submissive, and the creation or result.

The law of completion is present everywhere, in every form of life. The degree of its expression is forever advancing and rising toward perfection, from the lowest phase of physical manifestation to the highest plane of intellectual existence, where spiritual intelligence unites with its correlative feeling or emotion, and is expressed as dominant, life-giving power to heal and to restore. Occult philosophers of all ages have taught that by turning the passive, absorptive side of the mind toward the ever-present realm of activity or light, we must bring into being divine ideas, and this may be considered the purest form of healing.

In every person is this receptive nature and this absorptive principle; and such is the recipient capacity of the soul that it may receive and absorb all knowledge from the inexhaustible source of living Truth within the inner depths of the self, where priceless treasures of knowledge and wisdom are awaiting appropriation. Here the mystic principle of repose, which is neither sluggish nor inactive, is in control at the very center of activity.

The human soul is designed to be a recipient of divine nature and life. The "river of the water of life" is full to overflowing. When man removes the barriers that he has raised against it, when he holds his soul nonresistant and passive, divine love and wisdom will flow in, filling his finite spirit with its saving current. He will no longer need to depend upon outside influences and personalities, for he

89

will find that he has within himself a fount of living Truth springing from the infinite depths of his own being.

This passive faculty of the soul is a cardinal, vital power, but it attains mastery only through its union with the quickening power of Spirit. Just as a still lake among the hills mirrors the glory of the heavens above it, so passive substance reflects mental ideas. Without it no creation could be embodied or manifested. All created things are the expression of a principle that looks to intelligence as the power that gives form to thought. Outwardly expressed, the tendency is the unfolding of that universal purpose which ever seeks to embody itself in humanity.

Each person has been given the power to visualize the idea; nothing tangible can exist without the pre-existence of its spiritual source or idea; and thus we live, not from without, but from within outward. Having once gained a glimpse of our divine sonship and perceived the immortal self that can never be sick or unhappy, we try to externalize the divine idea in a material body. Turning the inner ear toward the "speaking silence" and becoming receptive to the mystic revelation, we shall receive the higher Truth of Being. Sincerely desiring to know and live this Truth, we turn the receptive side of our nature toward the world of pure intelligence and "in quietness and in confidence" passively wait for the quickening power of Spirit to vitalize and make us alive. Thus we come into a living communion with the infinite Christ principle.

Jesus practiced His method of healing through the divine alchemy of faith in this principle. Without this vital factor of faith the Christian religion is neither scientific nor practical and certainly not in accord with the teaching of its founder. Faith, Jesus taught, is the fundamental principle of healing, the very entrance of God Himself into the consciousness. Faith therefore is the first attribute we must receive, for without it we are spiritually dead and can do nothing. Through it we become alive to the Spirit and create true conditions.

Faith is spontaneity, vitality, the action of life. It is the assurance, the substance, of things hoped for, the conviction and evidence of things not seen. It is the power that links present with future, enabling us to stand on an impregnable foundation of Christianity. Jesus wasted no time or force in resisting and condemning outward conditions; He worked according to divine law and His faith gave Him mastery and dominion.

Through the exercise of faith Jesus made the

common people of His time great. He never blamed external conditions or depended upon them. Through faith alone He accomplished wonders. He believed it to be one of the highest powers of the soul, needing no aid; sufficient for all things and equal to all occasions. It fed the multitudes, healed the sick, stopped the mouths of lions, quenched the power of fire, turned to flight hostile armies, and raised the dead.

Through faith we may emerge into the four-dimensional realm, the inexhaustible, the cosmic consciousness. In this realm we shall perceive our spiritual perfection—of body, conditions, and environment. Through it we shall discern the universe of God and the truth of man. But it is useless to have intellectual conceptions that cannot be carried through to fulfillment. Every conception should register in an accomplished result. This is growth. As we gain the high vision there is born within us the impulse to act. Faith is the soul's vision, but unless it is acted upon it becomes ineffective, falling short of achievement.

In many of His parables the Master clearly illustrated the necessity of activity or "works," which is the Bible expression for accomplishment, manifestation, or demonstration of principle. Those who received the "talents" were required to use them. The wise "virgins" filled and trimmed their lamps. Many of those who were healed were instructed to do something. The blind man must "go to Siloam, and wash." The palsied one was instructed to arise, take up his bed, and go to his house. The man with the withered hand stretched forth his hand, and the leper was advised to go show himself to the priest, while those who would possess the "kingdom" willingly gave all they had ever earned in order to make it their own.

We are told that "faith apart from works is dead." This often occurs to me when people declare that they believe implicitly and pray faithfully to have their ills removed, yet they are not healed and their prayers remain unanswered. I invariably find that they expect their faith to restore them without effort or "works" on their part. They neglect the tangible half of vision, which completes the meaning of faith.

The spiritual faculty of faith can surmount any difficulty and banish every fear. It is a universal panacea which works miracles. You and I must each find it for ourselves—within ourselves—as a positive belief in the ever-present, ever-active, all-powerful Spirit of God, or good. Nothing matters but God and our attitude toward Him.

Next to the Nazarene, Paul stands out as the

most perfect type of a "faith" man in Bible history. In his letter to the Hebrews he produced a veritable "cloud of witnesses" from history to prove the efficacy of faith. Upon faith he based the accomplishments of science, invention, and exploration, the genius of leadership, the practical value of healing methods, and utopianism in social and economic relations. The quality he so lauded was to him a substantial expectation and a confident assurance of manifestation, a true combination of belief and trust.

There is something very contagious about Paul's absolute confidence and undoubting conviction, his bold firmness of mind; something that inspires self-confidence and self-reliance in us. We picture him as a true example of the faith doctrine that he preached so vehemently. On every side he encountered fear, inharmony, and trouble, yet he kept his faith in inherent divinity, remaining untouched by doubts, fears, and limitations.

It is possible to set a law in motion by faith and achieve miracles. Through faith we may "walk and talk with God" and clothe ourselves with His power. We are enabled through faith so to harmonize ourselves with the spiritual world that we can gain dominion over outer conditions. Faith may reign throughout the entire realm of nature when we understand that inner conviction or belief governs and controls the outer manifestation.

We are continually working according to the law that a belief held in consciousness must become manifest in outer conditions and circumstances. The law works "according to your faith," absolutely and irrevocably. Are you using the law constructively or destructively? According to your faith you receive. Have you placed your faith in sickness, failure, and poverty? Then you have received them. Have you placed your faith in the realities of life: love, substance, wholeness, truth? They are yours. Always you have had, and always you shall have "according to your faith."

Faith in eternal goodness is insight into the livingness of God. It fears no evil but confidently expects all good. It is adventurous and creative, and "believes" into visible expression the dynamic possibilities of the spiritual world. The secret of all healing is that the body registers the mind's belief in the perfection of man's powers and faculties as they are eternally existent in Divine Mind. According to your faith or belief in the imperfection or perfection of these powers, so shall it be unto you.

The Prayer of Faith

Prayer is a vast subject about which much has been written, for men have always prayed even though they have often lacked the spirit and understanding. However it has been and is misunderstood, prayer always has been and still is being woven into the very fabric of life. Its evolution has been curious, ever keeping step with humanity's advancement. Our intelligence is today demanding of it something practical: Does it heal and prosper us? Does it satisfy the deep desires of our heart?

Many years ago the apostle James wrote, "The prayer of faith will save the sick man." It is of this, the new yet very old thought of prayer as the basic foundation of spiritual healing, that I am writing. The true idea, expressed so many years ago, has been lost in a fog of misconception and misunderstanding. As time and understanding have come to interpret God as living principle rather than as anthropomorphic personality, prayer is no longer associated with supplication and beseeching. It is true that prayer has many forms, and I am aware that God is still approached as a powerful personage, vague and unseen, with cajoling flattery and explicit directions as to the exact method of consummating the favor requested. These specifications are often made with forceful persistence and "much speaking."

Prayer is no longer a cry to the Infinite from the finite; it is a science that depends upon principle. No person may presume to direct the Infinite by planning and specifying the manner in which his requests are to be answered. The answers must come in conformity with absolute law and often in ways beyond the knowledge or understanding of finite intelligence.

Prayer is a practical science and its rules must be learned and applied; if the conditions of application are not fulfilled, the answer is not obtained. Even our greatest scientists fail to get results until they develop a scientific method. Every law involves other laws, and their harmonious coordination insures perfect functioning. To know and comply with the laws of prayer is to get practical results, but the effective prayer must comply with orderly principle.

While it is not necessary that a person comprehend the spiritual significance of prayer in its every aspect in order to receive healing, it is essential that he be willing to be helped. Only such are ready for "the prayer of faith." Its efficacy is largely a question of erasing prejudices and anxious doubts from the mind, so that the healing energy of Divine Mind may have an undisputed right-of-way through the consciousness. Little can be accomplished through a barrier of unbelief or hostility. We know that even Jesus' power was limited by skepticism. At Nazareth He "did not do many mighty works . . . because of their unbelief."

Most people think they know how to pray, and they are hurt or indignant at the suggestion that their method is faulty. Many are continually asking why their prayers are not answered. They have faith, they declare; they ask, yet they do not receive. They "ask and do not receive" because they "ask wrongly." And this does not mean that some power called God has weighed their petitions and decided they should be denied. It means they have missed the right method of asking.

The first principle of the prayer of faith, as given by the great Teacher of prayer, was: "Go into your room and shut the door and pray to your Father who is in secret; and your Father who sees in secret will reward you." The door must be closed upon the noise and distraction of doubts and fears when one desires to commune quietly and alone with the Father, who dwells in the secret chamber of each individual consciousness. If one carries too many impedimenta in with him, the door cannot close, and therefore the turmoil continues. The "secret place of the Most High" can be entered only when human limitations are completely shut out. The "still small voice" can be heard only when you can "be still, and know."

The prayer of faith is agreement with God, not a plea to God to agree with us. If we make His way or will, which is always good will, our objective, we advance out of confusion into peace. In the eloquent silence of His presence there comes to us an answer to our turbulent questions, an assurance that He is good and that there can be no other power. There is only the good that has always been, that is now, and that always will be. We find then that our prayer of faith has not changed the plan of God or wrenched a favor from an unwilling giver. It has adjusted our limited ideas to the limitless capacity of the eternal purpose. It has translated His will into terms of accomplishment.

The first step in the prayer of faith that heals the sick is to establish a realization of the presence and power of God as infinite Mind, to whom "all things are possible" and who makes all things "possible to him who believes." This God thought, which is Truth—the Truth of Being—should enter and take possession of the mind and hold the consciousness. This is what is really meant by "holding a thought." However, it is actually the thought that holds the person, not the person who holds the thought. This Truth of Being is the Christ consciousness of divine sonship; the firm conviction that man was made in the image and likeness of perfection and has never been otherwise in divine consciousness.

We may think of prayer as "holding a thought" or "speaking the word"; as affirmation, concentration, or silent meditation; in whatever form we conceive it, it remains the basis of faith healing. There are those who, having reached a high place in spiritual intelligence, behold the divine self. These have been sufficiently "lifted up" to draw others unto them, above the plane of sin, sickness, and disease. Jesus, rising into the plane of the Christ or superconsciousness, opened gates of Truth along a shining way, through which heaven has been pouring its radiance upon the earth for nearly two thousand years.

Often the "spoken word," animated by a divine thought or a living truth, contains marvelous healing virtue. At the right time the right word reaches the inner life of man and makes him whole. It is possible that it may change the entire current and quality of a human life by carrying its message to some longing soul that is imploring, "Speak the word only and I shall be healed." It was thus that Jesus healed, condensing into the briefest sentences His inner life forces of faith and love and sending them forth as assertions or commands that reduced chaos to order and divine harmony. It was thus He restored bodies to wholeness. He used positive affirmations, never mental arguments. Those who know the Truth do not argue; they affirm.

I find that most people feel the necessity of dwelling in detail upon each ache or pain, magnifying its importance through repetition of symptoms. They fail to understand why recounting symptoms and labeling diseases is actually a hindrance to healing. The prayer that heals looks past all these to the positive realities of the life that is infinite and eternal.

Those who earnestly desire spiritual healing must resolve to put aside morbid, negative thinking and speaking, because detailed recitals of ailments emphasize conditions, giving them a specific place and influence in the consciousness. Many times they produce disorder where none exists and they aggravate a tendency to disorder if it does exist. The healing prayer of faith does not deal with symptoms or appearances of disease but with the realities of complete, harmonious living, which are health and wholeness and which cannot be impaired or lost. If you pray for health it will do you little good if you continue to groan and tell others of your suffering—if you keep on worrying about it, sympathizing with yourself and wanting others to feel sorry for you. How can health be manifested through you under such conditions?

Throughout my years of experience I have seen many so-called miracles come to pass. It is true, they have not always remained permanent, but I recall the great Master's comment regarding this: "Go, and do not sin again." It teaches me that a person is healed only as his thought is cleansed of error—or sin, as Jesus called it. Often the elimination of a single disturbing thought results in a cure, but unless there is established the spiritual health that springs from a conscious realization of the principle of life, through an awareness of the presence of God, the cure does not become established or permanent. It is like the seed in the parable of the sower which fell in stony places, springing up quickly but, because it had no root in itself, withering away when the sun shone scorchingly upon it.

Paul wrote to the Corinthians that the spiritual gift of healing had been extended to some. It does seem to be a natural endowment, but no person ever heals himself or another; even Jesus claimed no credit for the wonders He accomplished: "I can do nothing on my own authority." "The Father who dwells in me does his works." Yes, "the prayer of faith will save the sick man," *but* "the Lord will raise him up."

The prayer of faith realizes the perfection of faculties, not the perfection of the organs that express them. It begins at the beginning, at the source, entering the "holy of holies," the soul. Disease is repression working against expression. The man who was born blind did not come to Jesus asking for eye treatments. His prayer was, "Lord, let me receive my sight." Jesus was so conscious of the divine perfection of the faculties of the soul that He could free the imperfect beliefs of the afflicted ones who asked His help.

The healing prayer is a plea for the liberation of the soul's capacities and not, as many have been taught, a plea to God to withdraw the pain and suffering that He has inflicted upon us and that we must continue to endure, if it is His will. It has never been His will that man should suffer. "Thy will be done" is a plea for the absolute good will that is eternally seeking to express itself through you and me.

The healing prayer of faith is a perception of the "Lord's body," which is the true ideal in God consciousness. In every effectual spiritual treatment the entire attention must be turned toward the expectation of receiving the perfect God thought that destroys imperfect beliefs. Results will take care of themselves, for they must inevitably follow a change of thought.

Before anything can become manifest in physical form it must be created in the spiritual realm by thought. First the unseen and intangible, then the material and tangible. Thought is powerful, but it must be powerful and persistent in knowing the saving Truth that recognizes a celestial, undying self. There is an attitude of quiet confidence that lets God work through us; an eloquent stillness that ceases from contriving, from self-vindication, and from all expedients of wise forethought; a dynamic, expectant hush in which the soul may rest.

Jesus in performing His miracles of healing never

claimed any power or privilege that He did not recognize as belonging to all men. No one could be near Him without feeling the tremendous force of His mere presence. It inspired, encouraged, and healed all who came within its radius. It still dominates those who contact it in thought. We have all observed that certain individuals possess this healing presence, that their spiritual atmosphere is charged with a sanative contagion. There are medical doctors in whom mental influence is more important than any medicine they may prescribe. The influence they radiate is as much a fact in the mental realm as the perfume of flowers is in the physical world.

It is a matter of everyday experience that a negative, melancholy nature casts an atmosphere of gloom over those who are unfortunate enough to contact it. We all know too the beatific influence of a joyous, cheerful, positive presence and how its spiritual emanation blesses and enriches all who come within the range of its influence. Health and wholeness fairly flow forth from the one who possesses them.

Nothing exists that does not in some degree affect its environment. The tendency of all matter is to give out its energy. Therefore, "none of us lives to himself." You are not only receiving but sending out vibrations with every breath you take, every thought you think, every word you speak. You are continually giving something to everybody you contact. What sort of force do you emanate? Are you sending out vibrations that will be attracted by discouragement, sickness, and death? Or are they the sort that will harmonize only with happiness and health? Jesus drew His power from "on high," from the Father source of all energy. You and I may go to the same source, be quickened by the same Spirit, and send divine power forth in the same manner, for the healing of humanity.

The time to begin is now. Do not wait until some calamity comes upon you and you feel you must turn to spiritual healing as a last resort. Begin now to "lay aside every . . . sin [error] which clings so closely." Free your consciousness from those mental seeds which may develop into a harvest of troublesome growths. Resist the temptation to indulge in thinking and talking of sickness, calamity, and failure. Ask, seek, knock; you shall receive, find, and be admitted. Then have the faith to proceed in the face of all seeming difficulties, never doubting, always believing, that it will come to pass, that good will become manifest openly in your life as the expression of God.

Healing Your Financial Problems

There are just as definite laws governing the demonstration of prosperity as there are governing physical healing. To all who work in harmony with these laws no good thing is denied. Many a man is puzzled to find himself lacking supply when others, seemingly less intelligent, are able to accumulate wealth. Failure of any sort is due primarily to disregard of Principle, and those who are earnestly seeking reasons for their lack of abundance should inquire into the workings of divine law.

No mechanical invention exists nor any alchemy by which base metals can be miraculously transmuted into gold overnight. There is however an established principle with which to begin this transformation, and there is but one way and that is to discover the cause. I list this in the same category as that of physical distress. I know there are many who will disagree with me; those who are hesitant about trusting God with their material supply, although they willingly place their bodily ills and disturbed minds in His hands.

The old idea of poverty as some sort of virtue or divine trait of character must be abandoned. It is far from disgraceful to own few possessions, but it is certainly wrong to encourage a poverty habit of thought and to continue to lack either strength, good will, friends, or needful supply. Such expressions of spiritual ignorance are grave handicaps in the business of living.

Those who wince at the idea of associating God with material supply, as though such an association were blasphemous, are yet anxious to overtake fortune, even if they cannot bring themselves to connect it with anything spiritual. They must learn to know that opulence, properly understood, frees the spirit from hampering, demoralizing conditions of slavery to lack and want and is often an insurance against disease and crime.

People are usually disappointed when they are told the first step toward healing their finances. I know it is bewildering to be told that what underlies material manifestation is spiritual substance and that an abundant share of this must begin in mind; furthermore that it will not come by longing and wishing for money and the things money can buy, nor by concentrating on certain sums with which to pay bills or buy a home or give to charity; but rather by gaining a positive conviction of universal, infinite substance, which underlies all visible expression: the clear realization of God as the substance of the universe and therefore the substance of every human need.

We demonstrate only what we hold in consciousness, and when we image negative ideas in thought, they come forth and are manifested in our affairs. In like manner we establish a rich consciousness in the outer life. Abundance is demonstrated quickly when we have learned to live in the rich consciousness of a world of reality. Those whose activities lie principally in the domain of shifting human experiences are sure to be overtaken by the race belief in poverty and disaster.

All states of lack, limitation, and loss are mental states primarily and are prevalent because men have wandered away from the underlying principle of substance. These states are the outpicturing of pinched, dwarfed ideas of fear and lack in mind, and can be overcome only by thoughts that are fearless and positive. Some will take exception to the statement that lack is a spiritual blight; yet we know that it is a result of negative conditions in the mind and that the mental condition must be corrected before a manifestation of better things can be expected.

You may resent it as unsympathetic or ridiculous, but the fact remains that neither people nor conditions are holding back your good. The fault lies somewhere within yourself. There is no healing for you in the shaking, shifting conditions of human opinion. You have seen governments overthrown and political and economic panic take possession of men's minds. Things you once considered stable and permanent are swaying, tottering, and collapsing. You can never accomplish your security by joining in the discontent and discouragement surrounding you or by identifying yourself with anything that is perishable and changeable. And if you say it is impossible to ignore these conditions at a time when lack of supply is confronting humanity on every hand and continually presenting the unemployment situation, surely you must see that that is the time to seek a remedy. When both sociology and political economy have failed to point out any legitimate cause for the lack that holds the world in its clutches, why not search for it in the light of Truth?

The truth is that all lack of good is lack of God. Separation from God or good in the mental realm causes separation from good in the material realm. To realize this and through correct perception and constructive thinking to unite ourselves with God is to become one with the good that He is, the good that takes form in a truly permanent condition of healing: the good that reconstructs our affairs. We have learned that "faith apart from works is dead" as regards physical well-being; we must know also that believing *and* acting are necessary in achieving supply. In order to produce concrete results "works" must follow faith, in affairs as well as in the physical body.

Jesus taught continually that man is free from lack and want, that he need not be anxious or afraid. There is a tremendous need for the revival of the science that He practiced, for it covers all man's requirements and is a panacea for the impoverished condition that has come to be so emphasized in the consciousness of the race. To comprehend and practice the teachings of the Master would put an end to lack of whatever nature. To know that all the substance of God is ours is to cast off the sense of want and lift up the consciousness to the source of all good, thus reaching the very heart of infinite supply.

111

The Bible contains many promises of plenty for those who fulfill certain conditions. "Trust in the Lord, and do good; so shalt thou dwell in the land, and verily thou shalt be fed." "Be not . . . anxious for the morrow." "Seek ye first his kingdom . . . and all things shall be added." Jesus knew how to add supply whenever it was needed, yet He did not choose to burden Himself with the care of a great fortune. His advice on this subject has been widely misinterpreted as a disapproval of wealth. When He was asked by one who "had great possessions," "What lack I yet?" His reply was meant to emphasize the fact that things should not come first in the mind of their possessor.

The positive assurance of Jesus that "all things that the Father hath" were His made Him independent of the responsibility connected with the ownership of many "things." It is interesting to note that the prophets and teachers who were able to demonstrate supply at any time invariably chose simple ways of living for themselves. I do not wish to be misunderstood regarding this. The simple life of those days was far removed from the simple life of our time, with its comforts. Conditions are very different; civilization increases human needs. But "all . . . that the Father hath" is still ours to draw upon for all our needs.

Our problems have deep roots in our human consciousness, and the taproot, belief in lack, must be eradicated. Students often tell me that they find it simpler to demonstrate physical healing than freedom from "anxious" thought regarding tomorrow's supply. I know we find it easier to relax and trust in a higher power to restore physical health. I believe this is because we always to a certain extent subconsciously depend upon the body to right itself, with the aid of a vast reserve of natural strength, all of which appears to be lacking in the correction of impaired supply.

I realize too how extremely difficult it is to relax in the midst of clamoring bills and the crying needs of dear ones. Anxiety and worry hold the attention and blot out a vision of the infinite abundance that is always present to provide for those needs when it is confidently trusted. Consciousness of present lack and limitation causes mental tension and paralyzes the mind so that the stream of plenty cannot flow freely and naturally into manifestation.

One current creates another. Plenty must be in the mind before it can be realized in the material world. Constant concentration upon a diminishing bank account or an empty purse leads the mind to think of supply as a material thing and discourages the growth of spiritual abundance. Visualizing sums of money as appearing at certain fixed times limits both the supply of good and the time of its expression. Here again I know it is difficult to think constructively with lack and want staring one in the face. Yet it has been done, and what has been done can be done again by those who have the will to persevere.

Thought is the substance of all material things as well as the foundation of all that is spiritual. It is not one of a group of faculties; it is the essence of every mental activity, including all faculties, because it is the basis or foundation of them all. Things are thoughts made real, and the truer the thought the more perfect its actualized counterpart will be. Your world and its conditions are not going to change unless you yourself make the mental effort to change them by learning to think creatively, in terms that make for practical, constructive expression.

You have the power to choose your thoughts. Are you going to make them positive and constructive or negative and destructive? Negative thought, like disease, is fundamentally the result of ignorance. It is a contagious disease, but each person possesses the means of immunity in positive, constructive thought. You may banish forever your negative beliefs by putting other beliefs in their place. I grant you, this is not always easy, yet it is a simple process; and when you realize that it means the healing of certain conditions in your life, it should be an easy way to accomplish what you so earnestly desire.

It is dangerous to give way to mental enemies when you have the weapon of positive, affirmative thoughts with which to overcome them. Your beliefs feed upon your thoughts and feelings. When you withdraw the substance, they perish for lack of nourishment. As long as you feed your negative belief in hard times with thoughts of lack and feelings of fear it is going to "grow by what it feeds on." Thus you see how impossible it is to heal results without first eradicating causes.

The Bible is filled with "Fear nots" covering every situation and circumstance in human experience. Christianity provides man with an unfailing remedy for fear in its emphasis upon the protecting goodness that is always ready to sustain when it is thoroughly trusted. Fear leads its victim to the acute state of negativity known as self-pity. Its effect impoverishes its victims; for it checks true human sympathy because of the selfish concentration it expresses. One who views his own disappointments as unique personal misfortunes loses not only his own perspective but that of humanity as well.

The victim of self-pity invariably suspects people and conditions of being against him, and certainly that which he fears does come upon him. Through his own habits of thought he erects barriers between himself and the good that would otherwise reach him in the form of friends and opportunities. Even his prayer asks that his own will be done in the way he has planned it, without regard to the universal design. Because nothing comes his way he feels that his rightful deserts are being withheld from him, and each new disappointment convinces him that injustice is being dealt out to him. If he were told that the one thing he lacks is readiness to sacrifice his store of self-pity and belief in injustice, he would go away sorrowful, for he has "great possessions" along those lines.

Fear is also a relative of hoarding, and by hoarding I do not mean storing up money and hiding it away. Money can be hoarded even while it is being spent, through one's reluctance to part with it. It is the "cheerful giver" that is blessed in his giving, through release of mental tension, which opens up the supply channels. There are those who have great possessions yet who impoverish themselves by giving, because they cannot really "let go" of their material wealth. There are others, who seem to own very little, who enrich themselves by even the smallest expenditure, because they know that "the one base thing in the eternal scheme is to render no return," that there is some spending that they cannot afford not to afford.

Why is it that so many people are more concerned with getting than with giving? Wanting something for nothing and getting it, they fail to appreciate it. If riches are to bring us happiness we cannot obtain them by grasping and hoarding but by wisely using and generously giving that which we have.

There truly is an all-providing law of increase that, if complied with, supplies every need. Enough can never be said about the value of gratitude as an attribute in the manifestation of plenty.

Comparatively few have understood the working principle that lies back of praise and thanksgiving. We might study the Book of Psalms to great advantage in this connection. Underlying its lyrics there are laws of plenty. Whatever the poet's dominant theme may have been, each poem reaches a climax of ecstatic gratitude of spirit, not so much because of what God has done as for what He is; not because of what has already been manifested but because of what has been prepared for those who love and praise God.

Gratitude is much more than an emotional release; it belongs in the category of practical things. It is a force of accumulation, a positive motive force. Expressing it in praise and thanksgiving is a magnet whose power is to attract and increase everything it contacts. It is a liberation of spirit to which spirit responds, with results that tend to perpetuate themselves. Praise and thanksgiving are positive attitudes of mind, infallible solvents of those destructive forces which are creating your problems.

If you would solve your problems, remember that true appreciation of God's gifts is a recognition of your relationship to Him and to the limitless resources that you may contact at any time, in any place. Learn to give thanks in advance. Thanksgiving is a powerful remedy whose basic element is faith, faith in an eternal goodness from which all things proceed. Based upon this faith which anticipates the fulfillment of promised good, thanksgiving is bound to be accumulative. Magnetize your life with praise and let your daily meditation be "Father, I thank Thee."

Don't Let the Years Count

"How old are you?" It is a question we have grown up with from earliest childhood, and only recently have we begun to realize how incorrectly it has always been answered. It should have nothing to do with the number of years we have lived, yet we have been taught to measure them off and to divide them into Shakespeare's immortal "seven ages": infancy, childhood, youth, maturity, middle age, old age, and last of all, "second childishness and mere oblivion . . . sans everything."

We are coming to know that life is not measured by years but by states of mind and that the secret of youthfulness is in our own keeping. It lies in the viewpoint, the way of looking at life, the ability to let go of the past, to deal intelligently with the present, and to go forward confidently into the future. No person who has a sufficiently fine imagination need ever grow old, for he carries within himself the long-looked-for "fountain of youth" that Ponce de Leon sought so hopefully and persistently.

Growing old is a race belief, the result of erroneous, negative thinking. Every person has within himself the primal source of youth, which he may release and which will continue to flow as long as he feeds it from the inexhaustible font of Spirit, which "quickens" and makes alive. Life is a matter of going forward, and those who keep pace with its buoyant stride cannot grow old. You are only as old as your doubts and worries, your ideas and beliefs, your fears and despairs. The years do not count, for both youth and old age are states of mind.

We have counted the years and ages, and some have been older at thirty than others have been at ninety. There was once a prevailing idea that work should be laid aside somewhere in the sixties and that seventy was as far as one could reasonably expect to go. I am thankful for many exceptions to this fallacious delusion, for a number of witnesses to the fact that youth is of the mind and not of the calendar, for many proofs that listless idleness and retirement are greater enemies to life than work enthusiastically and intelligently done.

Neophobia is a word that means literally "fear of the new." It implies inability to adapt oneself to that which is different and modern, a dread of change from the old, prevailing order of things. It is a veritable sign of advancing age, and only the ability to adapt old ideas to changing conditions acts as a barrier to time, releasing the belief in those allotted "three score years and ten" which has become a fixation in the racial consciousness. A mind kept fresh and vital by a spirit of fervent enthusiasm and a desire for new adventure has found the secret of eternal youth.

The origin of the old-age concept is psychic rather than physical, and eternal youth is within the reach of anyone who cares to make it his goal and is willing to abide by principle. The first requirement is to let go of the outworn past and to look forward into the future with unfailing courage and interested curiosity; to greet each day as a new adventure, all the more thrilling because viewed from a perspective of passing years.

Why grow old? Surely no one wants to be left behind in this newest and greatest of all renaissances, when youth is the very spirit of the times; running riot perhaps but gradually readjusting standards and discarding ancient habits and traditions; stripping life of its camouflage and shams and substituting sane, sensible ideas. Youth is an expression of life, and life is eternal. Growing old even "gracefully" has gone out of fashion.

Walter Pitkin has emphasized the idea that life is only beginning at forty, once a day dreaded as the doorway to mental and physical decline—a fearful hazard to every man and woman. What a change has taken place in our world! Forty has come to be not a milestone but a signboard, pointing to richer, happier, and fuller possibilities of living; a time when tempestuous moods and emotions have grown calmer and one is able to "see life sanely and see it whole." Since the world has grown so complex, it requires rare ability to know much about it until one has reached the age of forty. Until then education and experience are preparatory, building up to the real purpose of life.

At forty, one is fortunate to have gained enough knowledge and experience to begin the actual business of living. There are people who have made themselves old at forty by their habits of thought. They are forty years "old" and dread each succeeding birthday anniversary. Birthdays should not be celebrated if they cannot carry the meaning the word implies: days of birth—new birth, rebirth! If we ask, as Nicodemus did of Jesus, "How can these things be?" the answer is still as elusive to many as that of the Master was to His contemporaries: "Ye must be . . . born of the Spirit."

We understand spirit to be mind and a birth of spirit to be a renewal of mind that so "lifts up" the body that it may have eternal life. There are scientific facts to support this belief of the comparative few. Causes of death are numerous, but science has never found a reason why people *must* die, or why the cells in their bodies lose their fresh, youthful vigor.

More scientists are agreeing that old age is unnecessary and that men should be able to renew their youth. There is no principle that limits life, for life is an endless process of growth. We observe frequent evidence of renewal in the natural world, and always from within outward. The fact that our body cells are continually renewed is a well-known fact. We once learned that complete renewal occurred every seven years; the renewal of certain cells is a matter of months. The process of growth is casting off wornout cells and building new ones continuously. Why should young cells be replaced by old ones? Or healthy ones by those deficient in energy? Cells are broken up, used, cast off and replaced. Nature has no rule for making them older and weaker as the years pass.

Through ignorance and wrong thinking we grow old according to the race belief. It is a habit, a state of mind. We grow old because we believe we must. Nature produces the body cells and we stamp them with our habits of thought, making them something nature never intended them to be. It is amazing to note how little interest mankind has taken in investigating the actual cause of cell deterioration.

What the mind images the body expresses. If the mind is kept fresh by a youthful spirit of courage and adventure, devotion to ideals, interest in new experiences, and adaptability to changing conditions, its owner has found the secret not alone of the emotional impulsive factor but of the organic as well. Whether our thoughts and beliefs are true or false, the body responds accurately to them. The true idea literally revitalizes the organism by replenishing its worn-out cells with fresh, new ones. The alarm clock of age need not unwind; it is our business to be so wide awake to the truth of life that we shall not need even the first tinkle that heralds its unwinding. After all, why should it be so incredible that a power which can create is just as able to recreate?

Life is a perpetual process of tearing down and building up. Potentially it has perfect balance, but human ignorance and error have interfered with its rhythmic equilibrium. Science has demonstrated the fact many times that thought controls the heart action and that it may direct and concentrate the circulation of the blood. Yet making these significant experiments practical has been slow. If it is thus possible to make the mind a definite factor in organic control, it is quite rational to believe that, applied to cell metabolism, it is man's key to eternal life. Traditional race belief is the great enemy of this radical new thought, and automatically stamps new cells with the negative belief.

Erroneous thinking continually binds and limits man's creation of his physical body, building into its cells weakness, poverty, old age, and death. His material body tends to deteriorate like any machine, but the difference is that the body has an inherent, automatic, and practically unlimited power of renewal. It is self-starting, self-building, self-operative, and self-renewing. A worn machine must be scrapped, but a worn body can be renewed and rejuvenated. The same power that devitalized its cells, through wrong thinking, can most assuredly build them up again.

A body does not wear out and fall into decay because of its age; nor do its various organs waste away in the manner that constant use wears out mechanical parts. The workman, swinging an axe all day, builds up his right arm and side to a greater muscular development than that of his left. If use causes deterioration, the opposite would be true. Unused muscles become flabby and often waste away altogether. The truth about the body is that man possesses an organism that should never wear out, although it often rusts out.

The materialists says that life *is* because the body exists. He adds that it is dependent upon food and drink for its sustenance and that it functions because it is natural for an organism to do so, and when its functioning power is exhausted it dies. It is true that food and drink are necessary conditions for the operation of life's forces, but the body must depend upon something more for its existence. The Master taught the true life principle: "Man shall not live by bread alone, but by every word that proceedeth out of the mouth of God." "It is the spirit that giveth life; the flesh profiteth nothing."

The engine works when power is driven through it; the power is the life of the engine. The body functions not entirely because of its organic mechanism but because of a live, invisible force radiating through it. Spirit is the life of the body. The engine's life, unlike spirit, cannot build the body through which it operates.

The mighty universal force of Spirit that we recognize as life is not altogether dependent upon material substance for its operation, yet it must have a body through which to function on the material plane. Such a body has been created, in the ideal. It has been endowed with self-starting, self-generating, and self-renewing powers. It draws from its environment the sustenance it requires, and its usefulness is a matter of the activity and care exercised in preserving its fitness and perfect functioning. Given vitality in the body, there is greater vitality in the life force; power depends on the condition of the body. You cannot trifle with the principle, deliberately violate the law, and expect the power to continue.

The life force sweeps through all alike. That of the mammoth is no greater or more abundant than that of the tiny insect. The force is incapable of expressing age. It has no physiological limit. We ourselves are responsible for the disease and destruction that block its passage through us. Health and life are in our own keeping. Our mental state determines them as it does the expression of youth or old age.

The will to live must govern the functions and operations of the body in order to make it resilient and healthful. Those who desire eternal youth must think health, speak health, and live health. Their mental attitude must exclude the counting of years as a means of measuring age. They must recognize the source of all life and call upon it for vigor and strength. Every live cell in the body is so much molten energy, continually being molded into shape by thought!

If we choose to furnish molds of age, weakness, and inefficiency, these are what we must expect to create in bodily expression. On the other hand, if we refuse to think in negative terms such as these and regard life as something eternal and indestructible, it should be possible to remain both mentally young and physically fit, indefinitely. Such a radical opinion is confirmed by a statement of Dr. Charles R. Stockard of Cornell University, who is quoted as saying: "I would hesitate to say that a man might not be kept as he is at the age of twenty-five for several hundred years. It is possible to arrest the development of the embryo; I see no reason why it should not be possible to arrest development at *any* time—at the age of twenty-five, for instance, when the human being is at the height of his growth."

The idea of old age is so indelibly stamped upon the human consciousness, that to think otherwise is considered ridiculous. Yet there are some who have not accepted the edict of disintegration but who believe that

"Of the soul the body form doth take,

For soul is form, and doth the body make,"

as Edmund Spenser wrote three hundred years ago.

And if you ask why more have not demonstrated the principle, you must remember that believing against the powerful race thought is difficult. Keeping the mind youthful and elastic is not as simple as it sounds. There is so much to discourage it; environment and experience combine to brush away its bloom. The mind is allowed to grow tired and fall into the rut of habit. New, changed conditions become harder to meet, the spirit of adventure and the zest for new knowledge grow dull, trivialities are annoying, work grows burdensome, and all of these things write themselves on the body.

Changes in the physical organism, supposed to indicate age, are symptoms, not causes. The cause is in the mind. If you grow tired of life, be sure the body will let down. If you meet life eagerly, the body will respond. Carlyle once wrote that the secret of genius is to carry the spirit of childhood into old age. It is a reminder of the Master's formula: "Except ye turn, and become as little children"; as little children, forgetting the things that are past and confidently living in the joyous, ever-present now.

Don't let the years count! Keep your keen interest in life and refuse to let your habits solidify. Guard against increasing sensitiveness, irritability, and fear. Learn to ignore petty annoyances and to remain calmly undisturbed by trifling irritations. Cultivate an eagerness for new knowledge and experience, always refusing to hark back to "the good old days." Have a soul-absorbing work that breaks down limiting barriers of your own life, your own family, and your own troubles, aches, and pains and extends outward into the universal.

Above all else, remember that Spirit does not grow old. You are one with Spirit. As you identify yourself with it you are "transformed, by the renewing of your mind," and you learn to say with the Psalmist, "So teach us to number our days, that we may apply our hearts unto wisdom."

The Beginning and the Ending

The Gospel story begins and ends with a Savior whose saving or healing power is the fulfillment of Christianity. His existence upon the earthly plane was of such importance that it divided world history into two sections and marked the beginning of a new era of time. He brought not only a revelation but a revolution of thought into expression. Although He lived in a world governed by soldiers, He taught peace. The great Roman Empire was proud and haughty, but He urged humility. Men were cruel, false, and deceitful, but by His every word and act He proclaimed, "Be true!"

It seemed an impossible undertaking, this cleansing and healing of humanity, this establishing of a kingdom in the souls of men by a revelation of the nature of God as love. Very early in His ministry

He began teaching and demonstrating an unheard-of-principle, the law of love. To love God was the first of those commandments so jealously guarded by the theologians of the day. It was also first in the doctrine of Jesus, but to love mankind, although second in position, was to Him just as important, and these two commandments constituted His simple creed and comprised the entire law.

We cannot study the fifth chapter of Matthew without realizing that love practiced as the Master practiced it renders all other law unnecessary because it fulfills all law. It is no wonder that the disciples caught the idea and made it the prime factor in their work, or that Paul wrote around it the most sublime love letter that has ever been composed. To the Corinthian church he tried to recommend a panacea for every trouble that can come to humanity. He concluded that only three qualities "abide," faith, hope, love, but the greatest of these is love.

Above all else, Jesus used His power to heal and elevate human life. He knew that when a person is weak and sick, when his body is racked with pain, he has little joy in life, even though he may possess every other means of material comfort. Today, even though men still kill each other for greed and gain, I am convinced that the law of love is advancing in human relations. There are many who have sensed the true meaning of the essential principle of the Master's teaching and who have touched its infinitely constructive possibilities; who have found that their experience of real happiness has come through their radiation of the divine love to those around them, through their unselfish service in alleviating the distress of the world.

To many it will seem strange and unusual to classify love as spiritual health, closely connected with physical wholeness. Few regard such an "intangible" thing as love as an attribute of bodily healing. But the metaphysician sees it as a divine radiation, whose release quickens the spirit, lifts the life forces, and promotes physical soundness. This idea should be easy to understand in this scientific age, when the universe is rapidly being reduced to a system of vibratory force.

Love is good will in action. It holds the universe together by its constructive, dynamic, unifying power. It is the great solvent of every limitation and every problem; the one power transfusing itself through infinite channels. Modern man has learned a great deal about power, its application and control, but he is just beginning to realize that it begins and ends within himself, in his own mind. As dissipated energy is wasted energy, it should be his object to control and apply his power to the business of living.

Nothing gives one a greater realization of the power of thought than the knowledge that power constantly responds to man's will and that man has the ability to draw upon an inexhaustible reservoir of active energy at any time and in any place. Every day science is making discoveries proving that infinite forces of vitality do exist that have just begun to be utilized. Waves and radiations are no longer confined to the laboratory; they are fast becoming factors in our daily living. Eminent physicians are recognizing them in connection with the body, agreeing that the symphonic harmony of health depends on certain mental and bodily rhythms to which man may adjust himself individually.

The modern metaphysician prescribes thought vibration much as the physician treats disease by applying various heat and light and other rays. But there is this difference. The metaphysician substitutes the primary elements of the "love spectrum," the various capacities of soul that must be used to work with God to allow His fullness of power to be manifested as a radiant expression of spiritual healthfulness. He well knows that when these inherent capacities are used the body must respond with a manifestation of the health that eternally exists.

Healing is a natural result of energy liberated by means of definite ideas. Health is, just as God is; it needs only the opportunity to reveal itself freely and fully as the boundless, changeless, irrepressible, ever-lasting life of God, through His channel of expression: mankind. God's infinite life is love—life and love are inseparable; for God is love. To be conscious of Him is to be conscious of love, and healing is the result of this consciousness of God. To live consciously with Him and share His life one must necessarily be a partaker of the divine nature, where all life begins and in which it should ever remain existent.

. Healing is making whole, and wholeness suggests restoration to an original, preexistent completeness. When we speak of being restored to health, we are acknowledging it as an original, natural state of being. According to Plato, "God holds the soul attached to Himself by its root." To be rooted in divine love implies nourishment, growth, life. Paul emphasizes this in his letter to the Ephesians: "that according to the riches of his glory he may grant you to be strengthened with might through his Spirit in the inner man, and that Christ may dwell in your hearts through faith; that you, being rooted and grounded in love, may have power to comprehend with all the saints what is the breadth and length and height and depth, and to know the love of Christ which surpasses knowledge, that you may be filled with all the fulness of God."

Paul is convinced that nothing, either "tribulation, or distress, or persecution, or . . . peril, or sword," can separate us from the love of Christ. He is "sure that neither death, nor life, nor angels, nor principalities, nor things present, nor things to come, nor powers, nor height, nor depth, nor anything else in all creation, will be able to separate us from the love of God in Christ Jesus our Lord." We may use it as the key that opens the door to peace and happiness here and to perfect understanding hereafter. Love will solve every problem, and nothing in this world or any other can cut it off from us; for love is the master key that unlocks every door. It frees the imprisoned self and releases the individual powers. It is the key to every situation, breaking down all limitation and opening wide the door of spiritual healing.

Every person believes in love, but many understand it only on the material or physical plane. I am aware that it is one of the most baffling, elusive words in our language, used to indicate affection, passion, philanthropy, friendship, good will, and all manner of likes. It is decidedly not the erotic passion so many poets and novelists make of it— supremely selfish in motive and conduct—but a quality of Spirit. Although so difficult to define, although it has been misnamed, misunderstood, and misapplied, it remains the greatest power in the world, the very essence of well-being. Its power is inexhaustible, its possibilities unlimited.

The love I am speaking of is not dependent upon anything in the outer; no person or condition need influence it. It is in itself a state of blessedness, because it is the essence of God and intimately connected with our life. Thought is the connecting link between it and the material world. Inspired by love, thought establishes higher radiations in the body, radiations productive of greater energy and more truly rhythmic.

The spirit of love crowds out of men's minds all sense of bitterness because of fancied wrongs; it sets aside all difference and opens wide the windows of the soul, letting the God within shine forth. If God is love, then love is all that God is. No person can love God without this love's outflowing toward all of God's children; therefore love is the constructive, unifying power that holds the universe together.

"A new commandment I give to you, that you

love one another, even as I have loved you." This was almost the last injunction given by the Master to His disciples, and practicing it was to be a mark of identification. "By this all men will know that you are my disciples." Thus His teaching and His work met in one brilliant focus: the love that is the only panacea for the strife and inharmony of life.

Christianity fails to measure up to its mission if it cannot keep this supreme commandment. The principle of principles, the principle above every other, is love, which expresses itself in unselfish good will. If all Christians wore as a badge this principle of their Master, there would be no clash of creed and dogma, no greed of conquest, no bitterness of resentment. The meaning of Christianity lies not just in joining a church or subscribing to a creed. It is not in simply tolerating your fellow creatures. It is in being so filled with the love of all life as to feel responsible for it.

I realize the difficulty of loving those who lie and cheat, the stupid and the ignorant, the cruel and the unkind. But if we can, as Jesus did, look beyond ignorance and vice, back of lack and ugliness, past all erroneous thinking to the Christ Spirit inherent in every human being, we shall discover, as He did, the true reality that is each person's birthright. Jesus not only talked of this,

He lived it. Recognizing the divinity of humanity, He loved and healed it.

There is no use in preaching love if we cannot practice it. Like a productive garden, man must yield his love for the benefit of others. He must give it out and relieve the lack that has fixed itself in the race consciousness and is expressing itself as evil conditions. For evil is a sense of lack. What is sickness but a lack of health, sorrow but a lack of joy, poverty but a lack of supply? Evil then is associated with lack, and lack is something that *is not*. Its opposite is goodness, wholeness, completeness, that which lacks nothing because it is all. If you would receive goodness, you must give it out as the loving service that desires to help others by making their burdens lighter.

The world, humanity, needs your services, and as you give them cheerfully and lovingly power gravitates to you. Loving service, this revelation of spiritual law that all can comprehend and apply, arouses new interest in the divine love that is God. To recognize this divine love is to make it a practical power in your life, for it is a constructive force, the secret growth. It makes spiritual healing the most normal thing in life, the natural answer to the greatest and most importunate demand of the world, freedom from bodily suffering.

It is a mistaken idea that God ever "allows" sickness or suffering or that His will stands between it and its healing. "Thy will be done" is the prayer that Jesus taught His disciples, but this does not mean that God wills sickness, sorrow, or suffering for anyone. God's will is eternally good will. We repeat that God is love. Even imperfect human love does not will misery or pain. How much greater is the desire of divine love to bless and heal! It is not God's will that man should break the law of life and bring suffering upon himself by branding his body with the race consciousness of disease and death. We must know God as the principle of eternal love, in which there is no recognition of evil or error. God is love and love is God, and our "dis-ease," both mental and physical, arises from our act of rebellion in seceding from that universal love which includes all knowledge, all truth, all blessedness, all life, the greatest of the things that "abide," the healing power that never fails—love.

In his "Symposium" Plato gives a comprehensive idea of the love that "fills men with affection, and takes away their disaffection, making them meet together [in brotherly comradeship] . . . supplying kindness and banishing unkindness, giving friendship and forgiving enmity, the joy of the good, the wonder of the wise, the amazement of the gods;

desired by those who have no part in him, and precious to those who have the better part in him . . . regardful of the good, regardless of the evil. In every word, work, wish, fear [it becomes] pilot, comrade, helper, savior. [It is the] glory of gods and men, leader best and brightest: in whose footsteps let every man follow."

In the words of the Master, who knew well the healing power of the love that is the fulfilling of the law, I end this work: "A new commandment I give to you, that you love one another, even as I have loved you, that you also love one another."

Printed U.S.A.   131-P-1248-20M-10-75